THE IKIGAI WAY

Pursuing Passion, Wellness, and a Purpose-Filled Life

by
Well-Being Publishing

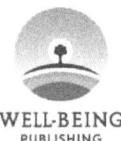

THE IKIGAI WAY

Pursuing Passion, Wellness,
and a Purpose-Filled Life

CONTENTS

EMBRACING THE IKIGAI JOURNEY

Embarking on the journey to discover one's ikigai is akin to setting sail towards a hidden yet immensely rewarding destination. The concept of ikigai—pronounced ee-kee-guy—stems from the Japanese language, where 'iki' refers to life and 'gai' translates to worth or value. It's a compass that guides individuals through the multifaceted maze of life, steering them toward a harmonious blend of passion, mission, vocation, and profession. At its core, ikigai is about aligning what you love with what the world needs, what you can be paid for, and what you're good at. But more significantly, it represents a philosophy that embraces the art of living, encouraging people to delve deep into their souls to discover a life filled with purpose and satisfaction.

In today's fast-paced, achievement-centric world, many people find themselves on a relentless pursuit of external validations. Yet, despite material success, a deep-seated void can still linger—a yearning for something more meaningful. That's where understanding your ikigai comes in. It's not simply a quest for happiness but a path to lasting fulfillment. It's an invitation to weave the threads of passion and practicality into a tapestry that is your life's purpose.

Imagine waking up each day energized, not weary of the tasks ahead, but enthusiastic about the opportunities to express your unique gifts. Such an existence might sound idyllic, yet it's entirely feasible when guided by the principles of ikigai. The journey offers no singular roadmap, as ikigai differs from one person to the next. However, the promise it holds is universal—an enriched quality of life marked by joy, resilience, and profound satisfaction.

This book invites you to explore the intersections where your talents meet your passions, where your joy spills into the lives of others, and where your work aligns with your heart's desire. It's a journey of introspection and action, of questioning and discovering, ultimately fostering a mindset that's both receptive and proactive. As you dig into these pages, you'll learn that ikigai is not a destination but a lifelong expedition, constantly evolving and reshaping as you grow and change.

More than just a personal pursuit, ikigai has rippling effects on those around us. By living in alignment with our purpose, we become beacons—shining examples of how a life infused with meaning can affect our communities and, by extension, the world. Engaging with your ikigai can foster meaningful relationships and create supportive networks where shared purposes amplify each individual's sense of fulfillment.

The practice of ikigai extends beyond the personal sphere into professional realms. In the workplace, understanding your ikigai could transform mundane jobs into calling-driven careers. It encourages the construction of environments where ambition coexists with well-being, ushering in an era where professional endeavors and personal passions intersect seamlessly. Businesses that harness the collective ikigai of their staff can redefine success not just in profits but in the enrichment of their workforce's lives.

Furthermore, ikigai serves as a foundation for resilience amidst life's inevitable challenges. In navigating setbacks, it's this purpose that morphs obstacles into learning opportunities, fostering a spirit of adaptability. Embracing change as a companion rather than a foe allows for continuous growth, bridging the gap between where you are and where you wish to go.

Ultimately, the journey to discover ikigai is a journey back to oneself. It's a reminder that within each of us lies a wellspring of potential waiting to be tapped. This book is your guide, offering wisdom, strategies, and exercises to aid in your personal exploration. Whether you're starting from scratch or looking to realign with a long-held purpose, these pages are crafted to support your quest for a life rich in meaning and satisfaction.

In opening yourself to the concept of ikigai, you invite transformation—not just in how you live but in how you perceive life at every turn. You're encouraged to explore, to dream, and most importantly, to be brave enough to pursue the life that calls you. The path may be winding and the discoveries sometimes unexpected, but therein lies the beauty of the ikigai journey. In fully embracing your ikigai, you step into a life of intention, where every day is aligned with your truest self. Let this journey guide you to an existence where passion and purpose merge, creating a symphony of enduring joy and fulfillment.

CHAPTER 1:
UNDERSTANDING IKIGAI

In the intricate tapestry of life, discovering one's ikigai—the profound sense of purpose that gives direction and meaning to our days—serves as a guiding star. Originating from the heart of Japanese culture, ikigai is more than just a concept; it's a harmonious blend of passion, mission, vocation, and profession. It embodies that sweet spot where what you love, what the world needs, what you can be paid for, and what you are good at converge. This balance fosters a life filled with satisfaction and continual growth, encouraging individuals to delve deeper into self-discovery and align their existence with the natural flow of joy and fulfillment. As you embark on this exploration, it's about finding that driving force—a reason to wake up with enthusiasm each morning. Ikigai is not just for individual gain; it's a path that enhances well-being, nurtures longevity, and cultivates a lasting legacy, inviting others to partake in a world enriched by shared happiness and purpose.

The History and Origins of Ikigai

To truly grasp the essence of *ikigai*, it's crucial to explore its roots. The concept of *ikigai* isn't just a modern-day philosophy or a trendy buzzword. Its origins stretch back to ancient Japan, interwoven with the cultural and historical fabric of the nation. Unpacking this tapestry of traditions and beliefs is essential to understand why this concept has resonated deeply with people across the world.

Let's start by examining the term itself. *Ikigai* is a compound of two Japanese words: *iki*, which means "life," and *gai*, which roughly translates to "worth" or "value." The combination suggests the worth or value of living. However, labeling it simply as "a reason for being" doesn't do it justice. It's so much more than a mere definition or a catchy phrase; it's a guiding principle that has provided direction for centuries. Instead of presenting life as a series of objectives to conquer, *ikigai* invites us to perceive it as a continuous flow, emphasizing balance and harmony.

The origins of *ikigai* can be traced back to the Heian period (794-1185 AD). This era was marked by cultural flourishment and a blossoming of Japanese literature, art, and philosophy. Noblemen and scholars were keen on understanding the nature of existence and what it means to live a good life. Philosophical discussions and writings from this time reflect an evolving awareness of personal well-being and fulfillment, aligning closely with the principles of *ikigai* as we know them today.

Japanese culture places a significant emphasis on community and the individual's role within it. The notion of *ikigai* naturally evolved within this context, where one's purpose was often tied to their contribution to the group. The intertwining of individual satisfaction with communal harmony reveals the intricate relationship between personal gratification and social responsibility. This dual focus helps explain why *ikigai* has a unique resonance that transcends mere personal satisfaction—it encompasses a larger social and ethical dimension.

Another layer to consider is the influence of Zen Buddhism and Shintoism. Both spiritual paths have deeply permeated Japanese culture, and they promote mindfulness, presence, and acceptance. Zen Buddhism, with its focus on living in the moment, cultivates an appreciation for everyday life. Meanwhile, Shintoism celebrates nature and the divine present in all things. Together, they provide a philosophical framework that supports the *ikigai* mindset—finding beauty and purpose in the daily activities that compose our lives.

Over time, *ikigai* has seeped into various facets of Japanese daily living, from art and education to work ethics and healthcare. It's not just about high-stakes decisions or transformative life changes; in fact, the practice of *ikigai* can be incredibly personal and nuanced. Whether it's the dedication to a craft, the joy of preparing a meal, or the commitment to one's family and community, *ikigai* expresses itself in myriad ways, reinforcing how purpose can be found in both profound and simple aspects of life.

Throughout history, regions like Okinawa have become celebrated examples of the *ikigai* way of life. This group of islands boasts one of the highest life expectancies in the world and is often studied for its correlation between well-being and longevity. Okinawans live by principles that reflect a deep sense of community and purpose. They engage in social activities, maintain close relationships, and continue finding purpose well into their older years. It's a testament to how *ikigai* isn't a static achievement but a dynamic way of living that evolves with each life stage.

As Japan entered the modern era, the power and applicability of *ikigai* transcended traditional boundaries. It wasn't confined to scholars or isolated to particular professions. Instead, it became a concept accessible to all, offering a lens through which anyone could view their life and choices meaningfully. In the post-war years, as Japan transformed into a bustling modern economy, *ikigai* assisted individuals in navigating the stresses of rapid urbanization, technology, and societal changes, reminding them of the timeless pursuit of a fulfilling life.

While its roots remain deeply seated in Japanese culture, the global interest in *ikigai* has surged in recent years. As modern life grows busier and more complex, people worldwide seek pathways to simplicity and joy—and this is where *ikigai* finds its wider appeal. People are yearning for a framework that helps balance the demands of career, family, and personal growth, making *ikigai* not just a cultural relic but a universal archetype for meaning and balance.

Ultimately, the history of *ikigai* is a beautiful narrative of how tradition interlaces with modernity, providing a philosophical compass that guides us toward a rewarding life. Understanding its origins offers more than just historical awareness; it offers a foundation upon which individuals can build their own version of a purposeful existence. Embracing *ikigai* means acknowledging the past, celebrating progress, and committing to a future where every moment holds potential and promise.

The legacy of *ikigai* isn't about imposing a one-size-fits-all purpose but inviting each of us to discover and embrace our unique paths, forging fulfillment through a balance of passions, contributions, and connection. This is its enduring power—an invitation to transform our everyday existence into something that doesn't just pass time but enriches and lengthens it with profound meaning. To delve into *ikigai* is to begin a journey, one that respects the past, engages the present, and inspires a fulfilling future.

Ikigai and Its Place in Japanese Culture

In the heart of Japanese culture, ikigai is more than just a concept; it's a way of life that seamlessly weaves purpose, passion, and perseverance into the fabric of everyday living. Rooted in the traditions of this island nation, ikigai serves as a guiding light that helps individuals navigate the complexities of life with grace and intention. It's not merely a question of finding what you love or what you're good at; it's about aligning those elements with what the world needs and what supports a sustainable life. This interconnection reflects an intrinsic balance that has been cherished across generations, illustrating why the Japanese often lead lives characterized by remarkable longevity and profound satisfaction. As we begin our journey to discover and nurture our own ikigai, we gain insights into living a fulfilling life that vibrates with meaning, helping us to embrace each moment with purpose and joy.

The Intersection of Joy, Fulfillment, and Longevity is where the essence of Ikigai truly comes alive in Japanese culture. It's that vibrant space where the laughter of the moment meets the serene knowledge of a life well-lived. It's not just about what keeps you waking up each morning; it's about savoring the experience throughout the entire day and carrying it into tomorrow. The Japanese have long understood that to lead a rewarding life, one must blend elements of joy, fulfillment, and longevity seamlessly.

At its core, Ikigai brings together these elements through a subtle and thoughtful arrangement of life's pursuits. It's not merely about living longer or amassing moments of happiness; it's about finding a balance that allows both to coexist and thrive. The Japanese notion of achieving a fulfilling life isn't driven by external ambitions alone, but rather through a harmony of internal alignment and outward expression. This involves a deliberate engagement with life's pleasures and challenges while being mindful of one's personal ethics and responsibilities.

Moreover, the sense of joy inherent in Ikigai isn't superficial. It's the joyful stirring that arises from engaging in activities that resonate with one's heart. This joy, lasting and resilient, is intertwined with purpose. The rhythm of daily life in Japan often embodies this interconnectedness, seen in practices like Hanami (flower viewing), which encourages a celebration of beauty in fleeting moments. By embracing transient joys, individuals are reminded of life's ephemerality and the importance of living fully in each moment.

Fulfillment goes deeper than simply ticking off goals. In Japanese culture, fulfillment is seen as the depth of meaning found in one's actions and relationships. It's about contribution rather than consumption, community rather than solitude. Roots of fulfillment stretch into nurturing connections with others and nature, which are integral to the Japanese way of life. The practice of Shinrin-yoku, or forest bathing, exemplifies this connection, providing a path to fulfillment through immersion in the natural world.

Longevity, in the framework of Ikigai, isn't merely about extending the number of years lived. Instead, it's about infusing the years with quality, and ensuring each one is abundant with experiences that matter. Okinawa, often referred to as the 'Land of the Immortals,' showcases longevity linked with Ikigai. The community lifestyle, rich with social interactions and purposeful endeavors, contributes to the remarkable lifespan of its residents. Here, longevity extends beyond physical existence; it embodies a life that continues to grow in purpose each day.

These three principles of joy, fulfillment, and longevity aren't isolated concepts in Japanese society—they're a way of life. By harmonizing these aspects, individuals create a personal ecosystem that encourages sustained happiness and health. The practice of Kaiseki, a traditional Japanese multi-course meal, is occasionally used as a metaphor for life lived according to Ikigai. Just as each dish is prepared with care and attention, so too should each life decision be crafted with the intent of nourishing both the body and soul.

Japanese culture beautifully illustrates the synergy that occurs when joy, fulfillment, and longevity intersect. This is seen in daily rituals that imbue routine actions with significance: the careful preparation of tea in a tea ceremony, the artful pruning of a bonsai tree, or even the deliberate steps of a morning exercise routine. By finding meaning and satisfaction in what might be perceived as mundane, the Japanese transform ordinary moments into extraordinary fragments of life's journey.

We might ponder how joy, fulfillment, and longevity weave into each person's individual tapestry of existence. Perhaps it begins with asking, "What feeds my spirit and keeps me eager to see tomorrow?" Aligning oneself with that question brings clarity to the pursuit of reason and contentment in everyday life. The intersection of these values within Ikigai serves as a potent reminder: to listen to our innermost desires, to act upon them with intention, and to accept the passage of time as an ally, rather than an adversary.

Thus, reflecting on the intersection within Ikigai implores us to examine our own lives—finding that sweet spot where joy, fulfillment, and longevity naturally converge. It's about crafting a life that's uniquely ours, a beautiful and intricate dance between our desires and our duties. Embracing this balance could unlock doors to undreamt destinies, paving the way for not just living, but truly thriving.

The Japanese culture, with its informed practices and deep respect for life's myriad facets, offers a blueprint for achieving this equilibrium. However, the journey is personal, requiring each individual to embark on their path to discover what brings them joy, what fulfills them, and how they can cultivate longevity. Perhaps the secret is in the conversation between these elements; a dialogue where life is cherished, lived, and shared in its fullest expression.

CHAPTER 2:
THE FOUR PILLARS OF IKIGAI

Understanding the four pillars of ikigai is pivotal to unlocking a life brimming with purpose, satisfaction, and joy. These pillars—What You Love, What the World Needs, What You Can be Paid For, and What You Are Good At—guide individuals in bridging passion with purpose, practicality with enrichment. They offer a scaffold to identify how personal passions align with global demands, transforming mundane existence into an exhilarating odyssey. By evaluating these dimensions, one can forge a harmonious balance where strengths meet opportunities and fulfillment dances with financial sustainability. Through weaving these elements into the fabric of daily life, ikigai not only becomes a pathway to purposeful existence but also a catalyst for continual growth and resilience in an ever-evolving world. So, let these pillars be the beacon that illuminates your journey, propelling you towards a destiny rich with meaning and vitality.

What You Love: Passion as a Compass

What drives you each morning to rise from the comfort of your bed? For many, the answer lies not in obligations or routines, but rather in passion—the kind that sets your soul on fire and propels you forward. Passion acts as a compass, steering the direction of our lives toward fulfillment and joy. In the context of Ikigai, the concept of loving what you do is vital because it forms one of its foundational pillars. To truly understand this pillar, we need to unpack what it means to find and follow passion as part of our journey toward purpose.

Think about a time when you were completely engrossed in an activity you adore. Maybe you were painting, playing an instrument, or even tinkering with engines. Hours slipped by unnoticed, and it felt effortless. This deep-seated enthusiasm is more than just interest—it's a passion, an intrinsic motivator that doesn't hinge on external rewards. In moments like these, we find a piece of our Ikigai, that enchanting harmony where what we love aligns with purpose and vitality.

Discovering what you love isn't always straightforward. It requires introspection and can be experienced at any age or phase of life. Often, societal expectations or familial pressures steer us away from uncovering our true desires. We might bury them beneath the layers of practicality or survival instincts. Despite these challenges, it's crucial to dig deep and explore different interests. List activities that excite you, professions you admire, or hobbies that you've always wanted to try but never did. Being curious and exploratory is the first step toward passion discovery.

There's a philosophical notion suggesting that when you do what you love, you'll never work a day in your life. While this may sound idealistic, there's truth in it. Passion transforms work into a delight rather than a burden. It energizes you rather than drains you. Yet, it's important to recognize that even passion-driven activities can have mundane moments. The magic lies in the consistent spark that keeps you going despite those less glamorous times. Pursuing what you love doesn't mean a life free of challenges; it means overcoming obstacles with an enthusiasm fueled by passion.

Imagine building your life on a foundation where passion is central. It leads you to construct a reality filled with joy and satisfaction. When passion guides you, decisions become clear. Career paths, personal milestones, and daily choices align with your inner desires, reducing friction often experienced when living out of sync with one's true interests. This alignment can lead to personal growth and open up opportunities previously unimagined. It's as if you're in tune with the universe's rhythm, your actions a natural extension of your core self.

Still, passion in isolation isn't sufficient. For passion to serve as a true compass in your Ikigai journey, it should intersect with the other pillars—what the world needs, what you can be paid for, and what you are good at. These interactions form a crucial balance that sustains and nourishes passion. For instance, perhaps you adore writing. This passion can be nurtured into a career, like journalism or authoring, that not only fulfills you but also meets society's needs and rewards you financially. The synergy of these aspects ensures a vibrant, balanced life.

Reflect on the impact pursuing passion has on mental and emotional health. Engaging in activities you love provides a natural escape from stress and contributes to deeper life satisfaction. People often report feeling happier and less anxious when regularly engaging in passions. There's an inherent value in doing things just for the joy they bring, and often, these activities foster a sense of identity and personal worth that spills over into other areas of life.

Furthermore, pursuing passion inspires others and fosters connection. When you express enthusiasm for what you love, you naturally attract like-minded individuals and foster community. These relationships further enrich your Ikigai, providing shared joy and encouragement. Imagine the bonds formed over shared passions— from book clubs to sports teams to artistic collaborations. Through these connections, passion becomes a powerful social glue, binding people with common interests and complementing the individual pursuit of purpose.

To harness the power of passion, it's essential to set aside time for your interests, even amid mundane obligations. Consider creative ways to weave passion into your everyday routine. Can you spare an hour a week to paint? Or perhaps volunteer on weekends doing something you love that benefits the community? Finding ways to incorporate your interests regularly reinforces their importance and offers balance to life's other responsibilities.

The journey toward a passion-driven life isn't always smooth. There might be sacrifices or tough choices along the way. However, by consistently aligning actions with what you love, the rewards far outweigh the struggles. This dynamic path, constantly recalibrated by passion, leads to a life rich in fulfillment and meaning. It nudges you away from complacency into a world of possibility, offering a sense of purpose that fuels each day.

Finally, as we explore passion's role in guiding us, remember that the quest is ongoing. Your passions may evolve, grow, or even change entirely over time, and that's perfectly natural. This fluidity is where the beauty of living through your passion lies—ever-changing, ever-new, always ready to take your life in fresh, exciting directions. In the great journey of Ikigai, let passion chart your course, forever acting as your personal compass toward a life well-lived.

What the World Needs: Finding Your Contribution

Amid the tapestry of life, your unique contribution is a thread that weaves through, connecting your personal journey to the broader world. This section of discovering your ikigai, what the world needs, invites reflection on how you can offer more than just your skills or passions but provide what the world genuinely requires. By aligning what you contribute with global needs, you don't just find your purpose; you craft a legacy of impact.

Understanding what the world needs with deep observation. The world is a complex canvas filled with problems and possibilities. What societal challenges stir your soul? Is it climate change, socioeconomic inequalities, or perhaps the quest for mental health awareness? Your ikigai is not solely an internal pursuit; it's a call to engage outwardly with empathy. Often, identifying these needs is the first step to understanding where you might fit within the puzzle.

It's not uncommon to feel overwhelmed when contemplating global needs. Yet, this sense of enormity shouldn't daunt you. Instead, it should energize you to carve out a niche where your contributions can shine. Remember, no single person is expected to solve the world's problems alone. The enduring impact is built on collective effort, with each individual adding their piece to the larger mosaic. Small actions, when accumulated over time and across communities, lead to substantial change.

Finding your contribution involves self-exploration and the courage to ask difficult questions. What injustices or gaps exist within your community? How can your talents or passions address these? Think small and local. Often, change starts from home. Perhaps you're an artist who can raise awareness through thought-provoking imagery, or a teacher inspired to develop new methods for engaging reluctant learners. Even seemingly modest contributions can ripple outward, sparking broader change.

But where to begin? Start by listening, truly listening, to the world around you. This involves immersion in conversations, perhaps volunteering, or simply being present in diverse environments. With attentive presence, you'll witness first-hand the wants and needs of those around you. This approach not only broadens your perspective but also enriches your understanding, allowing your contributions to become more intentional and aligned with genuine demand.

It's also crucial to harmonize your actions with your values. When what you offer resonates with both your personal values and external needs, your work will feel more meaningful and enduring. Values act as a compass, guiding you through the uncharted, often tumultuous terrain of life. This alignment ensures authenticity in your contributions, enhancing both personal fulfillment and societal benefit.

Your contribution might not follow traditional paths. In our interconnected world, the shapes and forms of solutions are as varied as the challenges they address. Artistic expression, technological innovation, grassroots activism—all serve as potential pathways. Embrace the unique qualities that make you, you. The diversity in contributions creates the robustness needed to face multifaceted global issues.

Reflect on historical figures who have made significant impacts, often starting with small steps. Think of those who challenged the status quo with unconventional ideas that subsequently transformed societal landscapes. They didn't just identify what the world needed; they acted decisively, often incrementally, but always persistently. In their stories, you may find inspiration—that ordinary individuals, imbued with extraordinary resolve, can indeed change the world.

This journey of contribution is deeply personal yet profoundly universal. What you offer becomes a testament to your life's work, a legacy preceding you. Therefore, approach this with both gravity and lightness—understanding the responsibility and the joy in it. When you uncover not just a need but *your* need to serve that cause, you've tapped into a vein of ikigai that infuses life with unparalleled meaning and satisfaction.

In sum, as you engage with this pillar of ikigai, know it's less about grand gestures and more about sincere, intentional commitment to the needs you identify. Keep asking where you fit within the world's needs, and be earnest in your pursuit to serve them. It's in this endeavor that we find not only our deepest fulfillment but also contribute to writing an enduring chapter in the human story—one built on interconnectedness, understanding, and a shared desire for a better world. Through these efforts, step by step, person by person, we edge closer to a world where our collective ikigais illuminate and enrich every corner of life.

What You Can be Paid For: Aligning Profession with Purpose

It's not just about the paycheck. Sure, the financial aspect is crucial when it comes to choosing a career path, but what if you could find a way to earn a living that also feeds your soul? This is where the third pillar of Ikigai kicks in: What You Can be Paid For. It's about finding that sweet spot where vocational interests and financial sustainability meet, crafting a career that resonates with who you are at your core.

The pursuit of professional purpose can often seem daunting, yet it begins with a simple but profound question: What skills do you possess that others are willing to pay for? This isn't merely about leveraging your resume or job history but tuning into those tasks and roles that truly make you feel alive while simultaneously meeting a market need. When your work aligns with your values and strengths, what you do daily becomes an integral facet of your identity. It transcends the transaction of time for money.

Some people find their calling early and set out on a straight path toward it. Others, however, stumble across a multitude of job titles, scattering skills across different industries like breadcrumbs along a twisting trail. If you belong to the latter group, take heart. This journey infuses you with versatility, contributing to a rich tapestry of experience that might just be your competitive edge. Each role teaches something valuable, and often, those lessons reveal unexpected ways you can contribute to the world. The key lies in trusting the process and remaining open to where your unique combination of skills might lead you.

This purposeful alignment is especially significant when we consider the constraints of time. You spend a large portion of your waking life working, so why not make it meaningful? The hours spent at your job should ideally echo your passions and values. It brings to mind the idea of *shokunin*, a Japanese term for the art of being a craftsman. Whether you're a software developer or a barista, infusing mindfulness and dedication into your craft elevates it from mere task execution to the creation of something profound.

Consider this: We are part of an interconnected system. While it's important that your professional efforts support you financially, it's equally crucial that they create value for others. Reflect on the balance between giving and receiving in your current professional scenario. Are you providing something that is not only of value but also genuinely impactful? When your work enhances others' lives, it propels you toward a purpose-driven existence where professional validation goes beyond monetary recompense.

In today's fast-paced, hyperconnected world, many individuals find themselves trapped in careers that sap their energy rather than renew it. The daily grind can easily become a cycle of exhaustion and disengagement. Identifying and transitioning into work that excites rather than drains you is essential. Start small but think big. Imagine the kind of work that doesn't just compensate you adequately but ignites a passion within you. This vision could encompass anything from becoming a consultant who dictates your own hours to an artist whose works inspire global audiences.

Remember, aligning profession with purpose doesn't mean chasing grandiose dreams immediately if it's not viable. It's perfectly okay to start where you are while keeping your aspirations at the horizon. Perhaps you can expand on a current role to encompass more duties you genuinely enjoy. Alternatively, consider side projects where your passions align more closely with career goals, offering a test ground and potential stepping stone to future endeavors.

Disruption is a potent catalyst for career evolution, so remain vigilant for opportunities that challenge your current state. These moments often present themselves through unexpected job offers, project shifts, or even during periods of doubt in your own career path. Lean into them rather than shying away. They hold the seeds for meaningful transformation. Emerging technologies, shifting economic paradigms, and burgeoning industries could serve as catalysts for innovation within your chosen field, revealing new avenues to explore professional alignment with purpose.

Lastly, the financial aspect must be approached pragmatically. We all have bills to pay, and there is dignity in every job done with integrity. Yet, it's worthwhile to explore ways to redefine what financial success means. Is it merely a paycheck, or can it be the surplus of time, flexibility, and joy obtained from a job that matches your values? Financial planners often advise setting medium- and long-term goals instead of simply thinking from one paycheck to the next. Apply this mindset to your career and forge a path toward a fulfilling role that financially sustains and enriches your life.

When you align what you can be paid for with your greater purpose, your work becomes an extension of your ikigai—a harmonious cycle that not only nurtures your wallet but also your spirit. It's a journey worth embarking upon, and along the way, you might just discover that fulfillment isn't a destination but an ever-evolving process. You become not only the architect of your financial future but the craftsman of your legacy.

What You Are Good At: Harnessing Personal Strengths

In our quest for ikigai, understanding and capitalizing on what we're good at is a fundamental step. It's part of the intricate dance of self-discovery, where we joyfully embrace our unique abilities and potential. So, what exactly does it mean to harness one's personal strengths? At its core, it involves recognizing your talents, nurturing them, and aligning them with your life's purpose. Here, we delve deep into why this pillar of ikigai is crucial, and how we can leverage our strengths to lead fulfilling lives.

Finding what you're good at isn't always as straightforward as it seems. Often, our natural talents are hidden beneath layers of self-doubt, societal expectations, or simply a lack of awareness. Discovering these talents requires introspection and sometimes the courage to step outside your comfort zone. It's about listening to the whispers of your soul telling you what truly feels right and pursuing those inclinations. When you begin to understand your strengths, you're essentially unlocking a pathway that has the power to guide you to your ikigai.

Consider moments in your life when time seemed to fly by. Activities where you lost yourself entirely, only to emerge feeling more energized than ever. That's often where you'll find your strengths lurking. Such moments of flow are precious indicators, pointing you towards what comes to you effortlessly. Recognizing these experiences is the first step in leveraging your personal strengths. They serve as reminders of the activities that ignite your spirit and where your true potential lies.

Once you identify your strengths, the next step is honing them. Like a sculptor chiseling a block of stone to reveal a magnificent statue, you, too, must work on refining your talents. This process requires dedication, practice, and often a willingness to seek guidance or mentorship. For instance, if you're naturally gifted at communication, joining a public speaking group or taking courses can help refine that ability. This honing process doesn't just enhance the skill itself; it boosts your confidence and lays a stronger foundation for your ikigai.

But how do we ensure that harnessing our personal strengths serves our broader ikigai? It's crucial to align these strengths with a purpose. Without purpose, even the most refined skills can become aimless pursuits, lacking the depth and satisfaction that come when tied to meaningful goals. Think of your strengths as tools; forging them into instruments that serve a purpose can lead to profound fulfillment. Ask yourself: How can I use my abilities to contribute to my community or society?

This alignment often requires an open-ended exploration where curiosity becomes your guide. Experiment with new ways to apply your strengths. Test them in various scenarios—some might affirm your path, while others may redirect you to places you hadn't considered before. This is a journey of self-exploration with the potential to expand your understanding of what you're truly good at.

It's also essential to remember that personal strengths don't exist in isolation. They complement and sometimes challenge each other, creating a dynamic interplay that defines your potential. Embracing this can liberate us from perfectionism, allowing us to see setbacks or weaknesses as opportunities for growth, rather than failures. It's this mindset that transforms personal strengths from mere skills into powerful drivers for achieving ikigai.

Moreover, leveraging personal strengths also means maintaining a balance. While it may be tempting to focus solely on the areas where we excel, ikigai thrives when we nurture our entire being. This includes acknowledging areas where we may not be as proficient and being open to continuous learning. Stepping beyond comfort zones not only broadens your skill set but also enriches your ikigai with diversity and adaptability.

Creating a supportive environment that fosters the development of your strengths is equally important. This includes surrounding yourself with people who inspire you, challenge you, and encourage your growth. A network of peers and mentors can provide the critical perspective and feedback needed to refine and harness your talents

18

effectively. Sharing victories and learning from shared experiences can be one of the most rewarding aspects of this journey.

It's worth mentioning that harnessing personal strengths is not a one-time event. As we evolve, our strengths and interests may shift. Lifelong learning and adaptability are keystone philosophies of the ikigai process. Embrace changes as they come, and allow them to guide the evolution of your interests and skills. By doing so, you keep the journey towards discovering your ikigai vibrant and enriching.

Reflect on how your strengths can inspire others. When aligned with purpose, our abilities don't just benefit ourselves; they create ripples that can positively impact those around us. Whether through mentorship, service, or simply by being a role model, the way you harness your strengths can be inspiring, leading others to discover their unique paths to ikigai.

In conclusion, recognizing and harnessing your personal strengths is like unlocking the door to your life's purpose. It's a journey that demands introspection, practice, adaptability, and a willingness to contribute beyond oneself. As you walk this path, remember that your strengths are not static; they grow and evolve with you. Embrace them with both humility and pride, and let them lead you to the heart of your ikigai, where fulfillment and joy await.

CHAPTER 3:
THE IKIGAI MINDSET

The journey toward discovering your ikigai isn't just about finding passion and purpose; it's about cultivating a mindset that nurtures these elements. At its core, the Ikigai mindset thrives on a positive outlook, embracing change, and maintaining a zest for learning that fuels an enduring sense of wonder. It's about shifting your perception to view each day as an opportunity, embracing failures as stepping stones towards mastery, and understanding that growth is fostered through both triumphs and trials. This mindset involves striking a harmonious balance between what resonates within your soul and the realities of everyday life. By integrating these principles into your thought processes, you open yourself to a richer, more rewarding existence. It's a continuous cycle of introspection, renewal, and growth, leading to a life where purpose and passion aren't just lofty ideals but living, breathing parts of each moment.

Cultivating a Positive Outlook

In the heart of the Ikigai mindset lies a powerful yet often overlooked tool: the cultivation of a positive outlook. It's more than just an attitude; it's a lens through which we can view the world, enriching our journey towards finding our unique purpose and living a fulfilling life. For many, maintaining a positive outlook is not an inherent trait but a skill that can be honed and nurtured through practice, patience, and intentional effort.

Shifting one's perspective to embrace positivity doesn't mean ignoring life's challenges or pretending everything is perfect. Instead, it's about acknowledging difficulties and choosing to focus on possibilities rather than limitations. This mindset aligns beautifully with the principles of Ikigai by gently leading us toward a more balanced and harmonious life. By fostering positivity, individuals can enhance each of the four pillars of Ikigai, bringing passion, purpose, and joy more vibrantly into their everyday experiences.

One of the most effective strategies in cultivating a positive outlook is the practice of gratitude. Taking a few moments each day to reflect on what we are thankful for can dramatically shift our mindset. Whether it's the warmth of the sun filtering through our windows, the aroma of morning coffee, or the comforting presence of a loved one, these small acknowledgments can accumulate to transform our outlook. Gratitude encourages us to recognize the abundance already present in our lives, fostering an internal environment ripe for positivity to flourish.

Another cornerstone in building a positive perspective is the art of mindfulness. By anchoring ourselves in the present, we become more attuned to our thoughts and emotions, observing them without judgment. This awareness allows us to catch negative thought patterns before they spiral, providing an opportunity to redirect our focus towards more constructive and uplifting narratives. Mindfulness, often intertwined with meditation practices, helps us cultivate resilience, enrich our emotional well-being, and ultimately, bring a touch of calm and clarity to our faster-paced lives.

Reflection is also a vital tool. At the end of each day, consider what went well and where there was room for improvement. By framing experiences as opportunities for growth, setbacks lose their sting and turn into stepping stones. This reflective attitude not only fortifies our positive outlook but also helps uncover insights crucial for personal growth and aligning with our Ikigai. Embracing this process means we're always learning, always evolving, and always moving toward our better selves.

Surrounding oneself with positivity is equally crucial. Engage with people who uplift and inspire, those who emulate the joy and purpose you seek. Our environment, from the individuals we interact with to the spaces we inhabit, profoundly influences our mindset. Adjusting these elements can create a nurturing backdrop for positivity to thrive. Consider curating your own space with elements that evoke happiness and creativity, such as art that resonates with your soul or music that stirs your spirit.

Physical well-being can't be overlooked when discussing positivity. A healthy body fosters a healthy mind. Regular physical activity, nutritious meals, and sufficient rest play an integral role in how we perceive the world. A well-maintained physical state is like fertile soil for positivity to take root and grow, reinforcing the connection between our body and mind as they work in tandem to support our quest for a meaningful existence.

Moreover, language shapes reality. The words we choose, whether in conversation with others or in our internal dialogue, powerfully impact our outlook. Replacing negative phrases with positive affirmations can gradually adjust our mindset. Instead of lamenting a situation with "I have to," reframe it to "I get to." This subtle shift not only alters our attitude but also enhances our appreciation for the present moment.

A positive outlook requires cultivation like a garden. Patience, dedication, and the willingness to prune away what no longer serves us allow for magnificent blooms of joy and purpose to emerge. Each small step taken toward adopting a more positive view is a seed planted toward a joyful life that's deeply aligned with our Ikigai.

Finally, remember that setbacks will happen. They're an inevitable part of life. The secret lies in how we choose to respond. With a positive outlook, each challenge becomes a lesson and each struggle, an opportunity to demonstrate resilience and ingenuity. Embrace these with an open heart, and they'll, in turn, fill your journey with growth and fulfillment.

As you integrate these practices into your daily routine, incrementally, you'll notice a change. Positivity not only enhances the vibration of your entire being but also sets the stage for a life filled with purpose, wonder, and potential—all key elements of living your Ikigai. Cultivate this outlook with care, and witness as it profoundly alters the fabric of your existence, allowing you to weave a life both extraordinary and uniquely yours.

Embracing Continuous Learning and Adaptation

In the realm of the Ikigai mindset, embracing continuous learning and adaptation becomes not just an option but a fundamental necessity. Life is dynamic, filled with ever-changing circumstances that require us to remain curious and open-minded. As we journey toward our ikigai, our willingness to learn and adapt shapes our ability to thrive amidst change. Just as nature demonstrates resilience through its cycles, our personal growth flourishes when we seek new knowledge and adjust to new experiences. This adaptability not only keeps us relevant in a fast-paced world but also fuels our passion and purpose. By adjusting our sails with the winds of change, we unlock untapped potential and keep our spirits invigorated, allowing us to realign with our ikigai, no matter what life presents. Each lesson and adaptation reinforces the mosaic of our existence, inspiring us to continue pursuing a path that resonates with longevity and fulfillment.

Lifelong Curiosity: The Secret to Youthful Energy is more than a mere sub-section of "Embracing Continuous Learning and

Adaptation"; it's a vital key to harnessing the power of your inner child. Embracing a mindset of lifelong curiosity can keep the spirit ageless, invigorate your mind, and keep life's colors vibrant. We often hear about the boundless energy of youth; what if that energy isn't tied to age but to a sense of wonder? Curiosity is an elixir that fuels both our minds and spirits—pushing us to explore, learn, and grow beyond the confines of conventional thinking.

At its core, curiosity drives us to ask questions, to seek knowledge beyond what we currently grasp, shaping a dynamic, ever-expanding view of the world. This intrinsic motivation goes hand-in-hand with the Japanese concept of Ikigai, where purpose isn't rigid or monolithic. Instead, it's flexible—growing and adapting as we move through different stages of life, nurtured by our willingness to continually learn. This is where curiosity intertwines with Ikigai, serving as its kinetic force, propelling us to embrace new roles, opportunities, and challenges with both joy and tenacity.

Consider how children face the world. Everything is new—a puzzle to be solved or a mystery to unravel. They radiate curiosity, asking "why," "what," and "how" at every turn. This same childlike wonder can be cultivated throughout adulthood, allowing us to remain youthful regardless of the years that pass. Engaging with our curiosity can lead us to unexpected places—to discover new passions, develop new skills, and interact with diverse people and ideas that may reshape our path to purpose.

Take Steve Jobs's famous calligraphy course story as a parable about the power of curiosity. Who knew that his random interest would later revolutionize digital typography? It's a testament to how chasing our curiosities, no matter how abstract or unproductive they may initially seem, can yield unexpectedly fruitful outcomes. Curiosity-led exploration can reveal intersections that transform dreams into reality, aligning them with our sense of self and purpose.

It's important to recognize that lifelong curiosity isn't just about accumulating knowledge; it's about opening ourselves up to change and adaptation. In a rapidly evolving world where technological advancements and societal shifts reshape the landscape, the ability to adapt can greatly influence both personal fulfillment and professional success. Curiosity acts as a lubricant for adaptation—it encourages us to remain pliable, welcoming new opportunities and altering our paths to align with the evolving world without losing sight of our core values.

To cultivate this curiosity, start by being intentional about the information and experiences you expose yourself to. Read widely, travel if you can, engage in deep conversations, and question the status quo. As you map your path to Ikigai, consider what you're naturally drawn to—explore that without fear. Maybe it's a new hobby, a different career path, or even an untried dish. The willingness to seek, to learn, and to open yourself to different perspectives can spark a youthful vibrancy that feeds into every other aspect of your life.

Curiosity should also be seen as a communal affair. It thrives when shared, when ideas are exchanged, challenged, and built upon. Engaging with others, discussing diverse topics, and learning from those around you can amplify your own understanding and keep your mental energy high. Community discussions, workshops, book clubs, and forums provide a rich tapestry of ideas and experiences, further stoking the fires of curiosity.

On the philosophical level, remaining curious is a profound act of humility. It acknowledges that we don't have all the answers—that there is always more to learn, to discover, and to understand. This stance not only enhances personal growth but also deepens the connections we have with others. As we cultivate this openness to learn and adapt, we create space for empathy and compassion, qualities invaluable in forging lasting, meaningful relationships.

Furthermore, this approach enhances our resilience. When curiosity is a cornerstone of our mindset, challenges become opportunities to grow and learn rather than obstacles. The roadblocks in life become less daunting when we view them through a lens of curiosity, asking what we can learn and how we might grow from the experience. This process can lead to impressive grit and adaptability—traits essential for navigating the complexities of life with ease and enthusiasm.

In essence, lifelong curiosity is a compelling ally in the quest for Ikigai. It's about maintaining youthful energy by welcoming the mysteries and uncertainties of life with a heart eager to learn. When curiosity propels you forward, every day is imbued with a sense of wonder, and there's always something novel waiting to be unearthed. So, let curiosity be your guide as you venture relentlessly toward your true purpose, allowing it to shape a life filled with both youthful zeal and meaningful existence.

CHAPTER 4:
LIVING INTENTIONALLY WITH IKIGAI

Living intentionally with ikigai is about embedding purpose into the fabric of our daily existence, transforming every action into a reflection of our innermost passions and values. It's not just about setting lofty goals, but also about refining the art of small, deliberate choices that resonate with our true self. By grounding ourselves in rituals and routines that are aligned with our personal ikigai, we create a robust framework for a life of meaning and fulfillment. This conscious alignment of actions with purpose allows us to navigate life's complexities with a sense of peace and joy, inviting us to savor the journey rather than just the destination. The power of purpose-driven actions ignites a profound energy within us, empowering each of us to live not only longer but also with a richer tapestry of experiences and connections.

Setting Goals Aligned with Your Ikigai

Imagine waking up each morning with a deep sense of clarity about your day and the life you want to create. This clarity stems from knowing your ikigai—your reason for being. To live intentionally means not just identifying this purpose but aligning your daily actions with it. Setting goals that resonate with your ikigai bridges the gap between where you are and where you wish to be. It's about harnessing that inner calling and translating it into tangible steps that lead to fulfillment.

When you set goals aligned with your ikigai, you're crafting a blueprint for a life that's not only successful but deeply fulfilling. These aren't just arbitrary targets or resolutions made in haste. Instead, they are thoughtful intentions rooted in what truly matters to you. Your goals become a reflection of your passions, your strengths, and the difference you wish to make in the world. They lead you towards a path where joy and purpose dance in harmony.

Setting goals starts with self-reflection. Delve into what truly ignites your passion. Ask yourself what activities or pursuits make time fly by. These moments when you're fully immersed in an activity often signal the presence of your ikigai. Delve deeper into these passions and question how they can be interwoven with your personal and professional life. The process may not always be straightforward, but therein lies the beauty of discovery.

Once you've identified these passions, it's time to consider what the world needs that you can uniquely offer. Your contribution becomes all the more potent when it addresses a gap or fulfills a need around you. This means staying attentive to the world, listening to its unsaid calls, and responding in ways that are authentic to you.

Another essential component is examining how you can be compensated for your endeavors. While passion and contribution are pivotal, merging them with a sustainable livelihood ensures that your pursuit of ikigai is not an isolated bubble but a practical, sustainable part of your life. Look for intersections where your passion meets market demand and social needs, paving the way for goals that are not just purposeful but also rewarding.

Next, harness your personal strengths and skills. Reflect on your past achievements, and recognize the talents that allowed you to succeed. Set goals that leverage these strengths to further fuel your journey toward ikigai. If your ikigai feels slightly elusive because of skill gaps, view them as areas for growth. Embrace the mindset of an eternal student; life is an ongoing learning process, and every day offers a new opportunity for personal development.

Creating goals aligned with your ikigai involves more than mere contemplation; it requires action. Break down your long-term visions into smaller, manageable milestones. Use short-term goals as building blocks that gradually guide you toward your ultimate purpose. This step-by-step approach lessens overwhelm, and each achievement propels you forward with renewed vigor.

The path of ikigai encourages flexibility. Life is unpredictable, and being too rigid may lead to unnecessary stress. Remain open to adaptations and transformations. Your path may not look like a straight line, and that's okay. It is in the process of aiming for these goals that you learn and grow, sometimes discovering new layers of yourself and your purpose.

Embedding your ikigai into goal setting isn't just about achieving static endpoints. It's about an evolving journey of discovery and fulfillment. As your life unfolds, your understanding of your ikigai may change. Let your goals be dynamic, evolving in sync with your growing awareness and experiences. By doing so, you nurture a lifelong engagement with purpose.

Once you've set your goals, reflect on how they're aligned with your day-to-day activities. Ensure that your daily actions and routines support your aspirations. Integrate small daily actions that are consistent with your larger goals, but also leave space for spontaneity and reflection. This balance keeps you engaged with the here and now while continuously prompting you toward your vision.

Inspiration can be a powerful ally. Surround yourself with reminders of your ikigai and goals. Whether it's vision boards, journaling, or simply revisiting your goals regularly, keep the fire of your dreams burning bright. Remember, setting goals alone won't suffice—it's the commitment to them that turns dreams into reality.

Finally, don't travel this path alone. Seek the support of a community or individuals who resonate with your journey. Engage in conversations that challenge and renew your vision, keeping you grounded to your purpose. A shared commitment to purpose, with like-minded individuals, amplifies your resolve, enriching your pursuit of a life aligned with ikigai.

Setting goals aligned with your ikigai is an ongoing exploration of aligning your deepest passions with your life's mission. It's a commitment to living intentionally and passionately, making sure every step you take resonates with your true self. With each goal achieved, you're not only moving closer to your personal aspirations but also contributing to a broader tapestry of meaning and fulfillment that impacts both your life and the world around you.

The Power of Small Daily Actions

Living intentionally with ikigai isn't about grand gestures; it's the small daily actions that truly pave the path to a fulfilling life. Each day offers a fresh opportunity to make choices that align with your core purpose, gradually weaving your life's tapestry with threads of intention. By breaking down the seemingly monumental goals into manageable tasks, we empower ourselves to steadily advance in meaningful ways. This daily dedication helps nurture habits that transform dreams into reality, as these small actions accumulate and compound over time, creating an unshakeable foundation of purpose and joy. It's in these moments, often overlooked, where the essence of ikigai profoundly takes root, reminding us that the journey to fulfillment is crafted in the subtleties of everyday life.

Rituals and Routines: Anchoring Your Day with Purpose are fundamental to living intentionally with ikigai. As we've seen in the previous sections, the power of small daily actions can't be overstated. It's the seemingly mundane tasks, repeated with intention, that shape our lives and bring us closer to discovering and living our ikigai. When we engage in rituals and routines, we anchor ourselves in the present, allowing our purpose to guide us through the ebb and flow of everyday life.

Rituals serve as powerful anchors because they transform ordinary tasks into acts of intention. By setting a specific time each morning to reflect or meditate, for instance, you start your day aligned with your values and purpose. This can be as simple as enjoying a quiet cup of tea, savoring the aroma, and letting the warmth prepare you for the challenges ahead. It's in these small, deliberate acts that we find grounding.

However, not all routines have to be quiet or solitary. They can involve interaction and engagement with others, like sharing family meals or participating in group activities. These connections not only enhance our sense of belonging but also remind us of what truly matters. As we draw near to our families or communities regularly, we continue creating memories and establishing a shared sense of purpose.

Incorporating movement into your routine can also profoundly impact your sense of purpose. Physical activities, whether it's a morning jog or a gentle yoga session, awaken the body and clear the mind. Movement fosters a connection between the physical and the mental, harmonizing our energies and opening us up to new ideas and perspectives.

Another key aspect of rituals is their ability to foster consistency. Consistency, in turn, creates habits. Habits are where the magic of small daily actions is most prevalent. When actions are woven into everyday life, they become less of a chore and more of a natural extension of yourself. It allows you to focus on your ikigai without being distracted by a constantly changing routine.

Furthermore, routines offer a sense of predictability that can be particularly comforting in turbulent times. They give us a framework to follow when the world seems chaotic, providing stability and reassurance. By sticking to a routine, you reinforce a personal sense of order and discipline, which are necessary to navigate the unpredictability of life with resilience and poise.

Your rituals, however, should never feel like a burden. Instead, they need to be regularly assessed and, if necessary, adapted as your life evolves. Just like the nature of ikigai is dynamic and ever-changing, so too should be your approach to routines. Tailor them to fit your current circumstances, ensuring they remain relevant and inspiring.

When establishing new rituals, start small. It's often tempting to overhaul your entire day with a multitude of practices, but success lies in simplicity. Choose one or two areas where you feel the greatest need for improvement or fulfillment. Gradually weave new elements into your day, giving each its due attention until it becomes an ingrained part of your routine.

Consider documenting your routines and reflecting on them periodically. Writing down your rituals gives you a tangible record of your journey and helps monitor your progress. It's a way to observe the layers of purpose you're adding to your life through seemingly minute changes.

Ultimately, rituals and routines are personal and unique to each individual. There's no one-size-fits-all formula, as your ikigai is distinctively yours. Honor your journey by crafting rituals that resonate with your inner self. Embrace the freedom to experiment and discover what best aligns with your values and aspirations.

As we delve deeper into living intentionally with ikigai, let these rituals serve as your compass. They will guide you through daily challenges and opportunities, ensuring each step is taken with purpose and intention. Allow them to illuminate your path and deepen your connection to the life you desire to lead.

CHAPTER 5:
THE ROLE OF COMMUNITY IN IKIGAI

As we delve deeper into the essence of *ikigai*, we uncover the profound influence that community plays in guiding us towards a life rich with meaning and joy. In cultures around the world, individuals have long drawn strength, purpose, and joy from the bonds they share with others. When it's community that uplifts us, challenges us, and celebrates with us, our journey toward fulfilling our *ikigai* becomes a shared endeavor, not a solitary quest. The warmth of human connections adds layers of purpose, becoming the fabric that holds our aspirations and dreams in place. When we nurture these bonds, we plant the seeds of resilience and growth, empowering not only ourselves but those around us. In essence, our life's purpose finds its greatest expression when it resonates through the lives of others, creating an unbroken circle of giving and receiving. Strong, supportive relationships fuel our passions, and offer new perspectives, reminding us that while our quests for personal fulfillment are deeply individual, their impact is beautifully communal.

Forming Meaningful Relationships

At the heart of every meaningful community lies the tapestry of relationships that bind individuals together with shared purpose and understanding. Ikigai, as a concept, thrives within this context of interconnectedness, where individuals find their place not just within themselves but alongside others. Forming meaningful relationships isn't just a social nicety; it's a cornerstone of ikigai, enriching our lives with depth, support, and mutual inspiration.

Consider the moments of shared silence with a friend who knows you intimately, or the excitement of a collaborative project with a colleague who shares your vision. These relationships, forged in the crucible of time and experience, become conduits through which our personal ikigai can grow. They provide us with the empathy and insights needed to further uncover who we are and what gives meaning to our existence.

Relationships are dynamic and ever-evolving; they require nurturing and intentionality. Just as ikigai involves a delicate balance of passion, mission, profession, and vocation, forming meaningful relationships demands commitment, openness, and a willingness to invest time and effort. The investment in these bonds isn't just transactional; it's transformational, offering both tangible and intangible returns.

For many, the first step toward forming meaningful relationships is understanding oneself. Self-awareness lays the groundwork for authentic connections. When you're aware of your values, passions, and goals, it becomes easier to relate to others on a deeper level. This self-awareness guides you in choosing which relationships to invest in and understanding what you can bring to each interaction.

One of the great insights of ikigai is that we don't have to embark on our journeys alone. The right friends, mentors, and companions offer perspectives and support that we might never have considered. Whether it's celebrating our successes or weathering life's storms, the people around us shape our experiences and influence our pathways.

An essential aspect of forming meaningful relationships is communication. Open, honest, and empathetic dialogue lays the foundation for connection and understanding. It's about listening as much as speaking, about recognizing the needs and perspectives of others, and allowing them to influence and enrich your own life journey.

Imagine walking a path where every individual you meet becomes a potential teacher or fellow traveler. Recognizing the unique value each person brings to your life allows for richer exchanges. It leads to growth and mutual respect, nurturing an ever-widening circle of relationships that contribute to a collective fulfillment of ikigai.

To foster these meaningful relationships, one must be proactive. It often involves reaching out beyond one's comfort zones, exploring new communities, or diving deeper into existing ones. Joining groups with shared interests or participating in community activities can be a way to meet like-minded individuals, enhancing both personal and communal ikigai.

However, the process isn't always easy. It may entail vulnerability and the risk of rejection or misunderstanding. But, as with anything worth pursuing, the steps taken toward forming and maintaining meaningful relationships are steps toward a life filled with purpose and joy. These relationships invite us to be more present, more giving, and ultimately, more fulfilled.

Mindfulness plays a crucial role here. Being present during interactions—not distracted or half-hearted—engenders trust and appreciation. It's being conscious of the moment and the people in front of you, letting them know they matter, and that their contributions are valued.

Within the embrace of meaningful relationships, there lies the potential for shared ikigai. When individuals bring their unique purposes together, there's a synergistic effect. This collaboration can lead to community initiatives, social change, or simply a strengthened bond between friends or colleagues striving toward shared ambitions.

In conclusion, forming meaningful relationships is not just about personal happiness—it's about contributing to a larger community of well-being. The people we connect with echo into the larger narrative of ikigai, weaving a shared story of purpose and fulfillment. Just as a flame shared grows stronger, our shared ikigai illuminates our collective journey, making each step richer, deeper, and more inspiring.

In dedicating ourselves to this practice, we honor not only our personal paths but the threads that interlace our community, building a world where every individual is seen, heard, and valued. Relationships, therefore, are not merely accessories to our lives but essential threads weaving together the fabric of our existence, creating a tapestry of shared purpose, illuminated by the guiding light of ikigai.

Building Support Networks for Shared Ikigai

We thrive when we're surrounded by others who resonate with our purpose. As we grow in our understanding of ikigai and the profound role it plays in personal fulfillment, it becomes evident that community and support networks are not just helpful, they're essential. These networks are like fertile soil, nurturing our ikigai and allowing it to flourish, drawing on shared resources and collective wisdom.

In a world that often prioritizes individual achievement, it's easy to forget the simple truth that we are inherently social beings. Our connections with others help us navigate life's complexities. When you share your journey towards ikigai with a network, it magnifies your efforts and provides a safety net during challenging times. A support network can range from family and friends to colleagues and community groups, all contributing uniquely to your sense of purpose.

Imagine this: a community all buzzing with their own ikigai, yet interconnected through shared values and goals. This isn't just a support group; it's an ecosystem where each individual's purpose invigorates and inspires the rest. This environment encourages the exchange of ideas and perspectives, acts as a sounding board for new thoughts, and offers companionship in the face of life's inevitable hardships.

Building these networks begins with forming meaningful relationships, a theme we've touched upon in previous sections. But it also involves seeking out those whose life perspectives align with your own ikigai. These are the people who 'get' you, who understand your dreams and ambition, and who can offer both constructive feedback and encouragement. In building such relationships, it's crucial to engage in active listening. This means not only hearing words but understanding intentions, emotions, and motivations.

Shared ikigai provides immense potential for collective action. Consider how a band of individuals, each pursuing a similar purpose, might unite their efforts to create something far greater than what they could achieve independently. Volunteering in local community projects, joining clubs or societal groups centered around common interests, or even participating in online forums are ways to nurture shared ikigai. Each member brings their unique strengths and contributes to a robust, purpose-driven community.

By participating in these networks, you benefit not only from the tangible support they offer but also from exposure to diverse ways of thinking. Engaging with varied opinions forces you to reassess your beliefs and assumptions, leading to personal growth and the refinement of your own ikigai. It's a process as rewarding as it is enlightening, kindling curiosity and sparking creativity.

At times, though, you'll need to take the initiative to create these connections, especially when they don't form organically. Start by identifying the values and interests you want to share. Whether it's a love of nature, an interest in art, or a passion for teaching, put yourself out there. Host small gatherings, attend seminars, or join groups that align with these interests. Take steps to reach out and trust that others are seeking similar connections.

Moreover, it's crucial to imbue these support networks with compassion and empathy, serving as reminders of our shared humanity. Helping others reach their potential as they assist you creates a positive feedback loop that keeps the community vibrant and driven. Empathy acts like a glue that binds the group together, ensuring that everyone feels valued and understood.

True fulfillment through shared ikigai often means bearing the burden of another's pain as much as their joy. Finding your ikigai doesn't mean all troubles dissipate. Instead, those within your network help share the load. When you encounter setbacks, your community can provide perspectives and solutions that you might not have considered alone. They help you bounce back, more resilient each time.

In moments of doubt, the shared experiences of your support network act as beacons of hope, highlighting new pathways and possibilities. These encounters build resilience, hardening your resolve as you pursue your dreams. When other members of your community achieve breakthroughs, their triumphs fuel your enthusiasm and renew your faith in your journey.

Ultimately, shared ikigai takes the concept of individual purpose out of isolation and places it within the collective sphere, merging personal growth with communal success. Building support networks shifts the focus from solitary journeys to collective endeavors, where interconnectedness amplifies our purpose and achievements.

So, as you journey on your path to discovering and living your ikigai, ask yourself: who is walking this journey with me? Are you part of a network that not only supports but also challenges you to become better? Consider not just what you can gain from these connections, but also what you can contribute in the ongoing dialogue of shared purpose.

By fostering these meaningful relationships and developing these networks, you're creating a community where your ikigai—and theirs—can thrive. The process becomes less about the destination and more about the shared journey, making the discovery of ikigai richer and more rewarding for everyone involved.

CHAPTER 6:
THE IKIGAI DIET: EATING FOR LONGEVITY

In the journey towards a fulfilling and extended life, the Ikigai diet emerges as a harmonizing blend of mindful eating and wholesome nutrition, aiming not just to nourish the body, but to invigorate the soul. Rooted in simplicity and balance, this cultural gem is not merely a diet; it's a lifestyle that celebrates the art of savoring every bite. Imagine each meal as a sacred ritual, where food isn't just fuel but a celebration of life's abundance. By embracing whole foods and local produce, you participate in a timeless dance of flavors and nutrients, forging a connection to the cycles of nature. This practice gently encourages you to slow down, be present, and let go of distractions, inviting an intimate communion with every grain and green. If you align your eating habits with your personal ikigai, you'll find yourself on a path not just to longevity, but to a life enriched with purpose and vitality.

Principles of Wholesome Nutrition

In the pursuit of a long and vibrant life, the foods we choose to eat hold an unparalleled power. When we align our choices with principles of wholesome nutrition, we unlock not just physical longevity, but a deeper sense of fulfillment that nourishes the soul. These principles aren't just about vitamins or calories; they form a bridge connecting our bodies to the natural world, enhancing our connection to both community and self.

At the heart of wholesome nutrition is the celebration of simplicity and balance. In today's fast-paced world, it's easy to be tempted by convenience over nutrition, grabbing pre-made meals or fast food. Yet, the essence of wholesome eating asks us to pause, reflect, and reconsider the impact of our dietary habits. It encourages us to choose whole foods—unprocessed and natural—to fuel our bodies. These choices are not just about sustaining our physical selves but are rooted in respect for the earth, understanding that what nurtures the soil can also nurture us.

Consider how traditional Japanese diets, rich with vegetables, grains, and seafood, naturally embody these principles. There's a rhythm and harmony to meals that reflect the natural cycles of life. The inclusion of seasonal greens and locally sourced fish isn't just nutritionally wise—it's a form of cultural art that offers respect to the changing tides and harvests. In a sense, choosing such foods becomes a ritual, a daily practice of gratitude and mindfulness.

Yet, wholesome nutrition is not a rigid set of rules. It is flexible, adapting as our needs change. Such flexibility encourages us to listen to our bodies, to recognize the signals it sends. Cravings can tell us what nutrients we might lack, and energy levels can indicate how well our current diet aligns with our physical needs. This intuitive eating is about reconnecting with ourselves, fostering an inner dialogue that leads to greater self-awareness.

Wholesome nutrition also highlights the importance of portion control. It's not about restricting our plates but learning to savor what we do consume. In cultures where food is truly appreciated, such as in Japan, meals are smaller, and each bite is considered. It's an approach that counters overconsumption, teaching us to cherish each flavor, each texture, in harmony with our body's natural satiety cues.

Moreover, adopting these principles involves cultivating a diverse palette. By broadening our food choices with a variety of flavors and nutrients, we engage in a holistic form of self-care. This diversity boosts our microbiomes and strengthens our immune system, allowing us to thrive. Incorporating foods rich in fiber, healthy fats, and lean proteins, ensures that our bodies operate at their optimal capacity, warding off chronic diseases and enhancing our overall vitality.

Furthermore, cooking becomes a form of meditation when we delve into wholesome nutrition. By selecting our ingredients with care and preparing them mindfully, we engage fully with the present moment. This practice is soothing in its simplicity and offers a sense of calm in the chaos of daily life. The sights, sounds, and aromas become a symphony of sensory experiences, transforming the act of cooking into an act of love for ourselves and those we share our meals with.

It's also crucial to recognize the moral and environmental impact of our dietary choices. Wholesome nutrition demands that we be conscientious consumers, considering the sustainability of the ingredients we use. By prioritizing organic and ethically sourced products, we respect the interconnectedness of our ecosystems. Such mindful consumption reduces our carbon footprint and supports the livelihoods of farmers who work with rather than against nature.

Yet, wholesome nutrition can extend beyond what is on our plates. It invites us to savor the experience of eating, to fully appreciate the flavors and textures. Meals can become moments of meditation, times when we slow down, breathe, and immerse ourselves in gratitude for the sustenance before us. This mindfulness transforms eating from a rote habit into an enriching practice that feeds not only the body but the spirit.

Another important aspect is the social dimension of food. The connections we forge over meals are vital to our emotional well-being. Sharing wholesome food with friends and family nurtures a sense of community and belonging, reinforcing our ikigai. Meals become more than nourishment; they are a celebration of bonds, laughter, conversations, and shared stories.

The principles of wholesome nutrition encourage us to reflect on the broader impact of our eating habits—not just for personal health but in understanding our place within the global tapestry. The choices we make have echoes, affecting farmers, workers, and environments worldwide. As such, embodying these principles is a pledge towards solidarity and compassion in every bite.

By integrating these practices, we can transform our approach to eating, making it a cornerstone of our ikigai. Wholesome nutrition is less a diet and more a way of life, one that aligns body, mind, and spirit in a harmonious symphony. As we embrace these principles, we find ourselves walking a path that not only extends longevity but enriches each moment with purpose and joy.

Mindful Eating: Savoring Every Bite

The journey to a fulfilling and long life begins with cultivating habits that nourish both mind and body. One such habit, deeply rooted in the Japanese culture of Ikigai, is mindful eating. This practice involves an intentional approach to food consumption, cherishing each moment from the first bite to the last. It's not just about consuming nutrients for survival; it's about reveling in the symphony of flavors, the act of preparation, and the gratitude for the sustenance provided by nature.

Imagine sitting down to a meal, free from distractions. Your phone is silenced, the television is off, and your sole focus is on the plate before you. Each ingredient tells a story, from the ripened tomato that absorbed summer's sun to the grains of rice meticulously cultivated over months. Mindful eating asks us to pause and truly relish the experience. It transforms meals from routine refueling into a celebration of life.

Mindfulness in eating also serves as an opportunity to reflect on the origins of your food. Where did it come from? Who cultivated, harvested, or prepared it? Such awareness not only fosters a deeper connection to your meals but also invites you to consider the ethical and environmental implications of your choices. Supporting farmers who practice sustainable agriculture, for example, aligns your consumption with the broader principles of Ikigai—living in harmony with nature and honoring the world's resources.

Research suggests that eating with mindfulness can significantly improve digestion, reduce overeating, and increase satisfaction. When you slow down and chew thoroughly, you're allowing your body the time to properly digest, ensuring maximum nutrient absorption. This aligns with the holistic approach of Ikigai, where every aspect of life is interconnected—mindful eating influences not just physical health, but mental clarity and emotional well-being too.

You might wonder how to incorporate this into your daily routine, especially when time seems scarce. Start with small, manageable steps. Perhaps begin by dedicating one meal a day to this practice. Observe the colors on your plate. Notice the aroma. Taste each bite deliberately, and focus on the textures. Over time, these simple acts will become second nature, enhancing your relationship with food and turning daily meals into moments of introspective peace.

The Japanese term "hara hachi bu" profoundly encapsulates the essence of mindful eating. It advises stopping eating when one is 80% full, a principle practiced in Okinawa—famous for its high concentration of centenarians. It's an invitation to listen to your body, acknowledging the signals of satiety it naturally sends, allowing for moderation without deprivation.

Moreover, this approach encourages gratitude—a cornerstone of mindful living. Before beginning a meal, consider taking a moment to express thanks. Whether it's a silent appreciation or a shared prayer at a communal table, gratitude enhances mindfulness by shifting focus from mere consumption to the abundance life offers.

Mindful eating can also foster community connections, an essential element of Ikigai. Sharing meals with family and friends enriches the experience, transforming it into an opportunity for bonding and shared joy. These gatherings aren't just about the food itself, but the stories and laughter exchanged, the mutual support, and the nurturing of human connections.

As you practice savoring each bite, you might find an unexpected bonus: a renewal of curiosity about cuisine. You may be inspired to explore new recipes, discover different culinary traditions, or visit local markets. This enthusiasm nurtures a lifelong love of learning, a pursuit that keeps the mind vibrant and engaged.

Ultimately, mindful eating within the Ikigai framework is less about what you eat and more about how you eat it. It's an ever-evolving journey that resonates with the intrinsic joy of living. By embracing this practice, you're aligning with a profound philosophy of life that values presence, health, and harmony.

As you continue exploring the principles of Ikigai, let each meal be a gift you give yourself, an opportunity to commune with nature's bounty, and a testament to living intentionally. By savoring each bite, let it guide you towards a more fulfilling, balanced, and joyful existence.

CHAPTER 7:
IKIGAI AND WELLNESS

In this chapter, we explore the profound connection between ikigai and wellness, integrating body and mind into a harmonious synergy. It's more than physical health; it's about achieving a state where your mental, emotional, and spiritual energies align with your life's purpose. Discovering your ikigai not only brings clarity to your goals but also fosters a lifestyle that brims with vitality and fulfillment. Movement plays a pivotal role here—view it not just as exercise but as a celebration of living. When you see physical activity as medicine for the soul, you unlock a vibrant energy that ripples into every aspect of life. By engaging in mindful practices that tune both body and mind, you nurture a well-rounded wellness, enabling you to stride confidently towards your destined purpose. Remember, the heart of wellness through ikigai isn't found in relentless pursuit but in the joy of the journey itself, as each step unfurls new paths to enrich your existence.

The Synergy of Body and Mind

Understanding the profound connection between body and mind is crucial on the journey to discovering your ikigai. This unity is not merely a concept; it's a lifestyle, a harmony that allows us to engage more completely with the world around us. In many ways, the body and mind are like two dancers, moving in sync, each step affecting the other's balance and grace. When we engage both in a symbiotic dance, we unlock the door to true well-being and fulfillment.

The mind has an undeniable influence over the body. Thoughts and emotions can manifest physically, affecting everything from our posture to our health. Imagine the impact of stress, which can lead to a tense neck or a pounding heart. Similarly, joy and laughter might elevate our spirits and improve physical wellness. By nurturing this synergy, harnessing the power of positive thinking and emotional intelligence, we allow the body to flourish and invigorate our mental state.

The relationship is reciprocal. Just as the mind influences the body, so too does the state of our physical being affect our mental clarity and emotional health. Exercise, for instance, releases endorphins, often enhancing mood and reducing anxiety. Regular physical activity not only strengthens muscles but also sharpens the mind, fostering a more resilient and adaptable outlook on life. It becomes apparent that when we care for our bodies, our minds are rewarded with increased focus and resilience.

It's not uncommon to hear that "movement is medicine." That phrase holds a wealth of truth. Physical activity is a key element in maintaining this balance, offering us a natural boost, infusing energy into our days, and granting the clarity of mind needed to pursue our passions. Yet, it isn't necessary to engage in exhaustive workouts or rigorous sports. Simple, mindful practices like yoga or tai chi can be incredibly powerful. These practices not only enhance physical strength and flexibility but also cultivate a meditative state, allowing for a deeper exploration of self and purpose.

Cultivating the mind's potential to influence the body isn't limited to reducing stress or increasing happiness. It extends to practices that enhance cognitive functioning and emotional equilibrium. Techniques such as meditation, mindfulness, and breathing exercises serve as bridges to align the mind-body connection. These practices encourage us to pause, reflect, and breathe, even in the midst of chaos.

As thoughts settle and clarity emerges, we're more equipped to confront challenges with a calm and thoughtful mindset.

Nutrition plays an integral role in this synergy too. What we fuel our bodies with can directly affect how we think, feel, and perform. A balanced diet doesn't just keep us physically healthy; it ensures the brain has the nutrients it needs to function optimally. Foods rich in omega-3s, antioxidants, and vitamins help maintain mental acuity and emotional balance, offering a foundation for a more purposeful life.

This intertwining of body and mind calls for a holistic approach. Both aspects feed into each other, creating a cycle of wellness that's greater than the sum of its parts. As we work on building this synergy, it's important to remember that patience and consistency are our allies. Progress may feel slow, but each step toward balance strengthens our foundation and aligns us more closely with our ikigai—our reason for being.

In your journey to harmony, consider the traditions and wisdom from other cultures that have long understood this connection. From Eastern philosophies to Western practices, the global perspective on body-mind integration offers a rich tapestry of insights and techniques to explore. These perspectives remind us that while the pathways may differ, the destination remains the same: a life of purpose, harmony, and fulfillment.

Imagine waking up each day with a sense of purpose wrapped in a body that's energized and a mind that's at peace. This is the gift of understanding and nurturing the synergy between body and mind. It's a continual practice—an essential dance through life that guides us towards our true north. By embracing this union, we lay the groundwork for living not only longer but with more zest and meaning. It's not just about longevity; it's about experiencing life as a vibrant journey, every step enriched by the balance we cultivate within ourselves.

As you move forward, consider what practices resonate most with your personal journey. What steps can you take today to enhance the synergy of your body and mind? Remember, this is a personal endeavor—a dance only you can choreograph. Embrace the small victories; they're the building blocks of a fulfilling life. In these moments, your ikigai will grow clearer, leading you with confidence through the intricate dance of your unique existence.

Movement as Medicine: Incorporating Physical Activity into Life

The journey to finding your ikigai is enriched by the synergy between the body and mind. It's not just about what you do intellectually but how you engage physically that can have a profound impact on your sense of purpose and well-being. Many scholars and psychologists have long emphasized this connection, noting that physical activity isn't merely a way to keep fit; it's an essential component of a balanced life, acting as a catalyst for emotional and mental clarity. When we move, we energize, we heal, and, most importantly, we live intentionally through the rhythm of our movements.

Think of movement not just as exercise, but as a way of life. In many cultures, particularly in Japan, where the concept of ikigai originated, there's a seamless blending of daily life and physical activity. It's about incorporating movement into your daily routine in a way that feels natural and purposeful. You don't have to hit the gym for hours to reap the benefits; instead, think of small, consistent actions that align with your lifestyle. Maybe it's choosing to walk or cycle to work, participating in a lunchtime yoga session, or even spending some time in the garden. Each step, each moment of movement, serves as a reminder of the vitality and joy you bring into your life.

Research has shown that physical activity can reduce symptoms of depression and anxiety, improve mood, and enhance cognitive function. These benefits manifest because movement stimulates the production of endorphins, which are the body's natural mood elevators. By incorporating intentional movement into our daily lives, we tap into this powerful, natural source of wellness. Consider this not just as a treatment but as a preventive measure, a way to sustain a balanced state of mind.

As we incorporate physical activity into our lives, it's crucial to find activities that align with our passions and our unique sense of ikigai. The key is to search for forms of movement that bring joy and fulfillment, not just chore-like tasks. Do you enjoy the tranquility of morning stretches? Does your heart race with excitement on a hiking trail? These are the types of movements that call to our spirits, urging us to align our physical and mental energies more harmoniously.

Furthermore, physical activity often brings with it a sense of community and belonging. Team sports, dance classes, and group yoga sessions are more than just opportunities to be active; they're avenues to connect with others on a deeper level. Forming these connections through movement, we often find support networks that enhance our overall sense of belonging and satisfaction. This aspect of community, intertwined with physical activity, fosters a shared sense of purpose that resonates with the communal aspect of ikigai.

One of the most profound realizations is that movement is indeed a form of therapy. The learned rhythm of tai chi, the controlled grace of ballet, or the outdoor adventure of a long run are not just activities—they're meditations in motion. These practices allow us to connect deeply with ourselves, providing a space to reflect, to let go of what's weighing us down, and to embrace the simplicity of being.

Incorporating physical activity is not solely about the act itself but about changing your perspective on movement. It's about letting go of the limiting belief that movement is a punishment or a chore. Instead, view it as a celebration of what the body can do and a cornerstone for discovering more about yourself. Whether you're lifting weights or simply taking a mindful walk, let each movement speak to your soul, reminding you of your capability and strength.

While we strive for perfect routines, it's important to be compassionate with ourselves. There will be days when movement feels like climbing a mountain and others when it feels like a gentle breeze. The goal is consistency and intention, not perfection. Listen to your body and honor its needs—whether that calls for intensity or rest.

Ultimately, moving with purpose embodies the essence of ikigai. It's about celebrating life through the art of motion, recognizing that our physical existence is a profound gift. As we lace up our shoes, take a seat on the yoga mat, or dive into the pool, we're not just exercising; we're choosing life, happiness, and a deeper connection to our true selves.

The journey to well-being through movement is ongoing, adaptive, and deeply personal. As you explore integrating movement into your life, remember that it is as much a mental and spiritual endeavor as it is physical. Through this exploration, you stand at the vibrant crossroads of health and purpose, ready to embrace the full spectrum of life with vigor and grace.

CHAPTER 8:
IKIGAI IN THE WORKPLACE

In today's fast-paced world, finding ikigai at work isn't just about clocking in and out—it's about crafting a professional life brimming with purpose and joy. Imagine weaving your passions into your daily tasks, turning obligations into opportunities for growth and fulfillment. Whether you're drawing inspiration from a mentor or harnessing your strengths in a collaborative project, the workplace becomes a canvas where ambition and well-being dance in harmony. It's about finding that 'sweet spot' where what you excel at meets what the world needs, creating a ripple effect of positivity and productivity. Balancing ambition with well-being isn't just a goal—it's an ongoing journey towards work-life harmony, ensuring that professional success doesn't come at the cost of personal happiness. Embrace the idea that every challenge is a chance to align closer with your professional purpose, making Mondays something to look forward to with a spark of excitement and a heart full of purpose.

Crafting Your Professional Purpose

In the dynamic landscape of work, the pursuit of a professional purpose can transform the mundane into the extraordinary. It's not just about earning a paycheck or climbing the corporate ladder—it's about aligning your work with your deeper values and passions. This alignment, known in Japanese philosophy as "ikigai," creates a harmonious balance that fuels motivation and nurtures fulfillment.

Ikigai in the workplace starts with introspection. Begin by exploring your passions and strengths, asking yourself what brings you immense joy and where your natural talents lie. It's here, at the intersection of what you love and are good at, that you often find the seeds of your professional purpose. When you identify the skills that not only drive you but also serve a need, you can align them with professional pursuits that will propel you forward.

Once you've pinpointed your passions, the next step is asking yourself how these can benefit the world. This requires a perspective shift from self-focused ambition to a broader, more inclusive view. Think about the impact your work can have on society, the environment, or even just your local community. By doing so, you add meaning to your tasks and connect more deeply to the outcomes of your labor.

The practical aspect of crafting your professional purpose often comes down to finding work that pays the bills while aligning with your personal mission. Money is undeniably a part of professional life, but when you're solely focused on it, fulfillment can become elusive. Financial needs are not to be dismissed, yet pursuing them in conjunction with your passions often leads to self-satisfaction that pure financial gain cannot buy.

Ikigai pushes you to think beyond conventional career paths and consider a broader array of options. It challenges you to integrate your talents, passions, and contributions into a cohesive career strategy. Sometimes this might mean altering your current role by expanding its scope or seeking new opportunities that better align with your ikigai. Your professional purpose should be as dynamic as you are, evolving with new interests and demands.

The essence of crafting a professional purpose is not confined to individual benefit but expands to include a sense of belonging and contribution to something larger than oneself. This is possible when talent, passion, and socio-economic needs overlap, creating a space where work feels less like a chore and more like a purposeful endeavor. When you achieve this alignment, you're not just changing your professional life; you're also laying down the framework for a more integrated, fulfilling existence.

Navigating workplace challenges becomes more manageable when your work holds purpose. Adversity and stress are a part of any job, but when aligned with your ikigai, they're transformed into opportunities for personal growth and insight. As you persevere and adapt, you build resilience—a key trait for sustaining professional satisfaction and performance over the long haul.

Incorporating ikigai into your work life doesn't mean every moment's going to be perfect. Instead, it suggests that you'll find profound satisfaction more consistently, and you'll be able to tackle inevitable setbacks with renewed energy and creativity. It's about viewing your career through the lens of continuous growth, where each experience—good or bad—adds depth to your professional journey.

For many, redefining professional purpose might call for a deeper engagement with learning and adaptation. You may explore new fields or gain additional skills to better match your ikigai with the realities of today's ever-evolving job market. This lifelong learning approach is not just about acquiring fresh skills. It's about cultivating a mindset that embraces change as a natural, productive element of your overarching purpose.

Networking, too, becomes a potent tool in crafting your professional purpose. By connecting with like-minded individuals or groups, you can discover new perspectives and opportunities to manifest your ikigai. Building genuine relationships can lead to collaborations and projects that resonate with your purpose, providing both growth and satisfaction.

Ultimately, the pursuit of professional purpose through ikigai is an active, ongoing journey. It's not a one-time decision but a practice of intentional living in the workplace. By continuously asking yourself what you love, what you're good at, what the world needs, and where you can be remunerated, you don't just create a professional purpose—you craft a life enriched by meaning and joy.

As you move forward, remember that crafting your professional purpose with ikigai isn't just a goal—it's a path that shapes every step, decision, and moment of your working life. Embracing this path means opening yourself to possibilities, being willing to explore, and above all, cherishing the journey toward a more fulfilling professional existence.

Work-Life Harmony: Balancing Ambition with Well-being

In the pursuit of ikigai within the workplace, it's vital to navigate the delicate balance between ambition and well-being. The modern professional landscape often glorifies relentless hustle, equating long hours with success and commitment. But in striving for personal and professional fulfillment, we must recognize that true success encompasses more than just climbing the corporate ladder. It involves cultivating a lifestyle that integrates work with personal satisfaction and health. This notion, though simple in theory, demands introspection and a conscientious approach.

Consider the concept of harmony as a symphony, where each instrument contributes to a coherent and restful whole. If any one instrument drowns out the others, the balance is lost, and the music devolves into chaos. Similarly, in life, when ambition overshadows personal well-being, the imbalance can lead to burnout, resentment, and an overall deterioration in quality of life. Thus, striking a harmonious balance becomes a crucial task, ensuring that neither ambition nor well-being screams louder than the other.

Embracing work-life harmony entails framing ambition within the context of well-being. It's essential to regularly assess what drives us and what sometimes drains us, as understanding these elements can frame our professional journeys. It's not about abandoning ambition but rather reshaping it to coexist with a life that nurtures health, happiness, and fulfillment.

At the heart of this balance is self-awareness. Understanding our limits and recognizing when work begins to impede personal health or happiness is pivotal. Regularly checking in with ourselves about what we need to thrive can guide actions, inspire changes, and shape paths that align with our ikigai. Ask yourself, "Does this ambition serve my broader purpose? Does it enhance my life or merely fill my time?" These reflections can be profound, subtly shifting the focus from doing more to doing what matters.

Moreover, it's essential to cultivate resilience, learning to adapt when life's unpredictable currents demand it. Jobs change, life circumstances alter, and what once felt right may no longer hold the same joy or meaning. Embracing this fluidity allows us to realign our ambitions with our personal well-being continuously. This adaptability doesn't imply abandoning goals at the first sign of discomfort but rather tuning into our inner compass to adjust when necessary.

Integrating joy and relaxation into our professional lives is a significant component of this balance. By engaging in activities that excite and rejuvenate, we avoid the trap of monotony and enhance our capacity for innovation and problem-solving. Whether it's a quick walk, an engaging hobby, or moments of mindfulness mapped into our day, these practices fuel us with energy that filters into our work endeavors.

Good leaders and organizations recognize the value of promoting a culture that appreciates work-life harmony. When workplaces endorse policies and environments that respect personal time and encourage well-being (like flexible work hours, mental health days, or professional development that includes personal growth), they invite higher productivity and increase employee satisfaction. They create spaces where being present and invigorated matters more than simply being productive.

Ultimately, aligning ambition with well-being involves conscious choices and the courage to stick to those choices. It requires sometimes saying "no" to things that detract from our well-being, deserving the same dedication and effort we place on our ambitions. Indeed, finding equilibrium doesn't imply limiting our capabilities or aspirations but rather empowering ourselves to pursue and attain what really enriches our lives.

In this pursuit, stories from various cultures teach us that a life truly lived is one where the heart and mind travel in concert. Just as ikigai marries passion with purpose, work-life harmony binds ambition to well-being. The workplace, then, becomes not just a venue for career growth but a space where life takes meaning—a chapter in our broader narrative of a balanced and fulfilling life.

Harmony between work ambitions and personal well-being is an ever-evolving journey rather than a fixed state. As we continue to seek our ikigai, acknowledging this dynamic interplay ensures that we're not merely living but thriving, creating not just a life of success but one rich in quality and satisfaction.

CHAPTER 9: OVERCOMING OBSTACLES TO IKIGAI

Life is rarely a smooth journey, and the pursuit of ikigai is no exception. It's not about the absence of challenges, but how we rise above them with resilience and strength. Setbacks are inevitable, but each one is a chance to learn, adapt, and reinforce our commitment to our true north. The key lies in understanding that obstacles are not roadblocks but rather stepping stones that guide us towards a deeper understanding of ourselves and our purpose. Embracing change with an open heart and a willing spirit allows us to navigate life's unpredictable twists with grace and courage. By focusing on resilience and adaptability, we can not only survive these challenges but thrive because of them, ultimately enriching our path to ikigai with wisdom and experience.

Dealing with Setbacks and Challenges

When we embark on the journey to discover our ikigai—our unique reason for being—setbacks and challenges are inevitable companions. The path to fulfillment, like any meaningful journey, is rarely linear. It's filled with twists, turns, and occasionally, what seem like dead ends. However, it's through navigating these obstacles that we grow stronger and wiser. Understanding how to deal with setbacks is crucial to sustaining our pursuit of purpose and living our ikigai daily.

Firstly, it's essential to reframe how we perceive setbacks. Instead of viewing them as failures or signs to abandon our path, we should see them as valuable lessons. Every challenge offers an opportunity to learn and gain insight into ourselves and our desires. As frustrating as a hurdle might be, it provides a moment to pause, assess, and realign our actions with our deeper goals.

Embracing a growth mindset is pivotal. This mindset encourages us to view our abilities and intelligence as malleable, molding with each experience. When setbacks arise, a growth mindset reminds us that we can improve through effort and perseverance. By seeing challenges as stepping stones to development, we can transform adversity into an essential part of our narrative.

In dealing with life's inevitable challenges, resilience is your steadfast ally. Resilience isn't an innate trait but a skill honed over time through experience and reflection. It is the ability to bounce back from setbacks, maintaining focus on long-term goals despite short-term difficulties. Cultivating resilience involves practicing self-compassion, setting realistic expectations, and holding onto the belief that adversity is only temporary.

One practical approach to cultivating resilience is maintaining a strong foundation of self-care. This includes ensuring we're physically and emotionally well-equipped to face challenges. Regular physical activity, nourishing meals, and adequate rest play significant roles in fortifying ourselves against stress. Moreover, incorporating mindfulness practices like meditation or journaling can help maintain mental clarity and emotional stability.

Another powerful tool in dealing with setbacks is adaptability. Life's unpredictable nature demands a certain level of flexibility. Instead of rigidly adhering to a predefined path, we can embrace a fluid approach, open to the changes and opportunities that may arise unexpectedly. Flexibility allows us to adjust our sails as the winds of life shift, helping us stay on course toward our ikigai.

Reflecting on past challenges can also provide guidance and strength. By examining how we've overcome previous difficulties, we can identify patterns and strategies that have served us well. This reflection isn't just about recounting past victories but truly understanding the processes that led to overcoming obstacles. What did we learn? How did those experiences shape who we are today? Revisiting the past provides valuable insights that can be applied to current hurdles.

Furthermore, sharing experiences and seeking support from others can be instrumental. Our communities, be it family, friends, or mentors, often provide perspective and encouragement when we need them most. Engaging in open dialogues about our challenges can lessen the isolation we feel during tough times and provide new solutions or approaches we hadn't considered. It's a reminder that the journey towards our ikigai is not one we must travel alone.

It's also important to foster an optimistic outlook. Optimism doesn't mean ignoring life's challenges; rather, it focuses on the possibilities each situation presents. It involves looking for the silver lining and finding gratitude even in difficult circumstances. Practicing gratitude can shift our mindset towards appreciation for what we have, helping us remain motivated and hopeful.

The power of small successes shouldn't be underestimated either. When faced with significant challenges, breaking them down into manageable tasks can provide a sense of progress and accomplishment. Each small success builds momentum, encouraging us to keep pushing forward. Celebrating these milestones boosts our confidence and reinforces our commitment to our larger goals.

Lastly, patience is a virtue often required on the road to ikigai. Pursuing purpose is not a race; it's a lifelong journey that evolves with us. Our passions may shift, our strengths may grow, and the world's needs may change. Embracing this fluidity requires patience with the process and trust in the unfolding of our journey.

In conclusion, dealing with setbacks and challenges is an inevitable part of the ikigai journey. By cultivating resilience and adaptability, drawing on support networks, maintaining optimism, and celebrating small wins, we can navigate these obstacles with grace and determination. Setbacks are not roadblocks; they are integral parts of our developmental landscape, shaping us into the individuals we're meant to become. As we overcome these challenges, our sense of purpose and fulfillment only strengthens, bringing us ever closer to living our true ikigai.

Resilience and Adaptability in Pursuit of Your True North

Embracing your ikigai is a journey, not a destination. As you venture through life, chasing that almost ethereal sense of purpose, obstacles are inevitable. They come in myriad forms—unexpected life events, inner doubts, or societal pressures. Yet, these challenges need not derail your quest. Instead, they serve as crucial teachers on your path to discovering your true north.

Resilience is more than just a buzzword; it's the backbone of enduring pursuit. It's the ability to bounce back in the face of adversity, to take life's punches and keep moving forward. Imagine resilience as a river flowing over rocks. The river doesn't stop at the obstacle; instead, it finds a new path, carving its way with persistence and grace. When you face challenges, it's vital to cultivate this same spirit. Acknowledge the setbacks, but don't dwell on them. Learn, adapt, and keep flowing. This mindset helps you maintain the momentum in your pursuit, and over time, it becomes a core part of how you live purposefully.

Adaptability, on the other hand, ensures that you're not rigid in your approach. Life is in constant flux, and what worked yesterday might not be effective today. Consider adaptability as the flexibility of a skilled musician who improvises on stage, responding to the subtle changes in the room and the band. In pursuing your ikigai, adaptability allows you to adjust your sails rather than forsake the voyage entirely when the winds of life change direction.

The key to fostering resilience and adaptability lies in self-awareness. Understand your strengths and weaknesses. When you do, resilience becomes about leveraging your strengths to overcome hurdles, while adaptability allows you to transform weaknesses into opportunities for growth. This self-awareness is not a static understanding but a dynamic, ongoing dialogue with yourself.

Practically speaking, how do we build these traits? Start by embracing discomfort. Challenge yourself regularly—whether it's taking on a new project, learning a new skill, or stepping out of your comfort zone. Each moment of discomfort is a training ground for resilience and adaptability. It's like a muscle that grows stronger with each stretch and strain.

Moreover, reflect on past experiences where you demonstrated resilience or adaptability. What did you do well? What could've been done differently? Journaling about these experiences can provide valuable insights, helping you formulate strategies to apply in the future. This reflective practice not only reinforces what you've learned but also heightens your intuitive response to new challenges.

Community plays a pivotal role as well. Surround yourself with people who embody resilience and adaptability. Share your experiences, learn from theirs. Often, the very act of telling your story can illuminate solutions you hadn't noticed before. Community support acts as a buffer, providing diverse perspectives that spark new ways to tackle challenges.

The journey to your ikigai is also facilitated by cultivating gratitude. Amidst chaos, gratitude grounds us like the roots of a tree. When setbacks occur, reflecting on what we're thankful for can shift our focus from what's lost to what remains, providing a stable footing from which to leap forward.

Furthermore, it's essential to set realistic goals, breaking them down into manageable steps. This approach not only reduces overwhelm but also allows for adjustments as needed, embodying the adaptive mindset. Progress, however incremental, fuels resilience, reminding us that each step brings us closer to our true north.

Importantly, understand that vulnerability is not the antithesis of resilience. Instead, it's a companion along the journey, allowing us to be truly open to what life offers. Vulnerability leads to authentic connections with others and deeper self-acceptance, enriching our path to fulfillment.

Ultimately, resilience and adaptability aren't just strategies but become part of your story. They shape your narrative and forge your identity as someone who doesn't simply exist but thrives irrespective of circumstances. By embodying these traits, you carve a path toward an ikigai that's vibrant and sustaining.

In conclusion, remember that resilience and adaptability in the pursuit of your true north are not destinations. They're ways of being, qualities that infuse your daily life, enabling you to face the world's unpredictability with courage and creativity. As you continue your exploration of ikigai, these traits not only enhance your journey but also amplify the fulfillment you find in every step along the way.

CHAPTER 10:
IKIGAI ACROSS CULTURES

Ikigai, with roots deeply embedded in Japanese culture, has transcended geographical and cultural boundaries, offering a universal framework for finding purpose and fulfillment. Across the globe, individuals are weaving the essence of ikigai into the tapestry of their lives, each culture infusing its unique nuances and perspectives into the concept. In the hustle and bustle of Western societies, ikigai is being embraced for its holistic balance between personal passions and vocational commitments. Meanwhile, in regions like Scandinavia, known for their exemplary quality of life, ikigai resonates through their emphasis on community, nature, and simplicity. This cross-cultural exploration enriches ikigai, transforming it into a versatile tool adaptable to anyone's life context, irrespective of cultural backdrops. By understanding and integrating elements from worldwide perspectives, we not only enhance our individual searches for meaning but also create a shared language of purpose that binds us in our human experience. Whatever corner of the world we call home, ikigai whispers that life can be lived fully, with intent and joy at its very core.

Global Perspectives on Purpose and Fulfillment

As we journey around the world in search of purpose and fulfillment, we encounter diverse cultures that each offer unique insights into what it means to live a life of meaning. While the concept of *ikigai* is deeply rooted in Japanese culture, similar ideas echo across various societies, connecting with universal themes of purpose, happiness, and longevity. The pursuit of a life filled with meaning is a common thread that weaves through the tapestry of human existence and understanding how different cultures embrace this quest can enrich our own lives.

In Scandinavian countries, there's a concept known as *lagom*, which roughly translates to "just the right amount." This philosophy promotes moderation, balance, and contentment—key elements for a purposeful life. By embracing *lagom*, individuals strive to find harmony in their personal and professional lives, avoiding excess and living sustainably in tune with their environment. This approach encourages people to prioritize well-being over the relentless pursuit of material success, a sentiment that resonates with the essence of *ikigai*.

Across the globe in India, the practice of yoga has long been associated with self-discovery and fulfillment. Beyond its physical aspects, yoga offers profound insights into the human mind and spirit, guiding individuals toward a deeper connection with themselves and the universe. By fostering mindfulness and presence, yoga helps practitioners cultivate inner peace, clarity, and a sense of purpose, much like *ikigai* in its encouragement to explore one's passions and strengths.

In Latin American cultures, the concept of *bienestar* captures the idea of well-being through connection and community. Strong family bonds and vibrant social networks are central to finding fulfillment, as these relationships provide emotional support and a sense of belonging. This communal approach mirrors the importance of meaningful relationships emphasized in *ikigai*, reminding us that pursuing purpose often involves nurturing the bonds we share with others, enhancing our collective experience of life.

Over in Bhutan, the measure of national success isn't Gross Domestic Product but rather Gross National Happiness. This small Himalayan kingdom focuses on holistic well-being, emphasizing sustainability, cultural preservation, and spiritual health. By prioritizing the quality of life over economic gain, Bhutan teaches the world that happiness and fulfillment stem from more than financial prosperity; they arise from living in harmony with one's values and environment.

In Australia, the Indigenous concept of *Yarn* points to storytelling as a way to explore one's place within the world. Passing down knowledge through stories helps individuals connect with their heritage, community, and environment. This tradition underscores the importance of understanding one's roots and cultivating a sense of identity and purpose through shared narratives—a theme that echoes the introspective aspect of *ikigai*, as individuals reflect on their life's journey and contributions.

Through these examples, we see that while every culture has its approach to purpose and fulfillment, several universal truths emerge. Meaningful connections, balance, and inner peace are crucial components of a fulfilling life. The values of community and sustainability underscore the importance of aligning personal goals with broader societal and environmental considerations. When we integrate such values into our own lives, we're better equipped to find our true purpose and cultivate the happiness that naturally flows from it.

Against the backdrop of these diverse perspectives, we gain a broader understanding of what it means to lead a purpose-driven life. The distinct contributions from different cultures highlight the varied paths that can lead to similar outcomes: a sense of fulfillment and joy. What's remarkable is how each cultural wisdom, regardless of origin, aligns seamlessly with the principles of *ikigai*—a testament to the universal pursuit of a balanced, joyful life.

In today's interconnected world, understanding these global perspectives on purpose can foster an appreciation for the different ways people strive to create meaningful lives. The fusion of these diverse philosophies equips us with a richer toolkit for personal development, encouraging us to broaden our horizons and consider alternative strategies in our pursuit of fulfillment. By embracing this diversity, we can transcend cultural boundaries and create a more harmonious, purpose-driven life for ourselves and future generations.

As we continue to explore the notion of *ikigai* in a global context, the path to personal fulfillment becomes clearer. The cultural practices we've examined reveal that although the terminology and traditions may differ, the underlying goals remain consistent. A purposeful life is within reach for those willing to learn from the world's diverse cultures and incorporate these valuable lessons into their unique journey.

Ultimately, in seeking a meaningful life, each perspective helps us see our challenges and opportunities through a new lens. Our global perspective enriches our search for *ikigai*, inspiring us to draw from an intricate weave of cultural wisdom that creates a robust foundation upon which we can build our own unique sense of purpose. It emphasizes that the quest for fulfillment isn't a solitary journey—it's one that benefits from the collective wisdom of humankind.

Adapting Ikigai to Diverse Life Contexts

In a world that is constantly shifting and evolving, the beauty of ikigai lies in its adaptability across diverse life contexts. As individuals explore their unique paths to purposefulness, they find that the core principles of ikigai remain steadfast. However, the application of these principles can be as varied as the individuals themselves, influenced by cultural nuances, personal circumstances, and societal shifts.

Imagine a young professional in bustling New York City and a retired educator in a serene Japanese village both seeking fulfillment. Their environments, cultural experiences, and personal challenges differ drastically. Yet, both can tap into the essence of ikigai to shape their lives with meaning. By understanding and adapting to their contexts, they can weave a coherent narrative of purpose.

For many, the journey begins by recognizing the role culture plays in shaping their perceptions of purpose. In Western cultures, there's often an emphasis on individualism and personal achievement. Here, ikigai might manifest as a career that aligns with personal passions or as a mission to enact change in the world. Conversely, in more collectivist cultures, where community and familial roles are emphasized, ikigai may be found in nurturing family bonds or contributing to communal success.

Even within a given culture, personal circumstances will shape how one engages with ikigai. Consider a mid-career professional who, faced with redundancy, sees their purpose shift from career advancement to mentorship. By embracing the flexibility of ikigai, they can find fulfillment in supporting others, an endeavor that not only aligns with their skills but also serves a communal need.

Societal changes, too, demand an adaptable understanding of ikigai. In an increasingly digital world, new professions and lifestyles are emerging, challenging traditional notions of purpose. A digital nomad might find their ikigai in the fusion of work and travel, satisfying their love of exploration while contributing unique skills to the global economy. The digital age offers unprecedented freedom to define one's path, yet it requires a conscious effort to remain connected to the core tenets of ikigai.

Understanding the fluidity of ikigai is crucial for those navigating significant life transitions. A stay-at-home parent returning to the workforce, for instance, might initially struggle to reconcile their past and future identities. Yet by evaluating their passions, strengths, and the needs of the world around them, they can redefine their ikigai, transforming what may seem like disjointed life chapters into a cohesive, purpose-driven narrative.

For some, adapting ikigai to their life's context means confronting and embracing diversity within themselves. This includes accepting imperfections, acknowledging evolving passions, and allowing one's ikigai to grow alongside them. Such an approach fosters resilience, as individuals permit themselves to reinvent their purpose without fear of judgment or failure.

Communities can also play a significant role in shaping and supporting individual ikigai. By fostering environments where diversity of purpose is celebrated, communities can enhance collective well-being. Social groups, whether local or virtual, offer valuable support networks where shared experiences and varying perspectives enrich one another's pursuit of purpose.

Ultimately, adapting ikigai to diverse life contexts is not about rigidly adhering to a predefined path. It's about being open to change, reflecting on one's journey, and allowing personal and cultural contexts to guide the unfolding of purpose. This adaptability does not dilute the essence of ikigai; rather, it reinforces its relevance in an ever-changing world.

In a world marked by constant transformation, ikigai stands as a beacon of grounded balance and enduring purpose. While contexts may vary vastly, the reflection and pursuit it encourages remain universally meaningful. Through conscious adaptation, ikigai can be a lifelong companion, evolving alongside the individual to meet the demands of an unpredictable life journey.

CHAPTER 11:
IKIGAI FOR THE NEXT GENERATION

As we navigate the shifting landscape of the modern world, the call to instill the timeless principles of ikigai in the younger generation becomes more crucial than ever. By teaching children and adolescents the art of finding joy in purpose, we equip them with the tools to craft a life brimming with meaning and satisfaction. Encouraging them to explore their passions, understand their strengths, and identify areas where they can contribute meaningfully to the world will help shape empowered individuals poised to make a positive impact. Embracing ikigai, not just as a personal philosophy but as a collective mission, can guide the next generation toward a future where purpose and joy are intrinsic to their existence. This journey, while unique for each individual, creates a tapestry of interconnected lives driven by purpose, underscoring the importance of passing down this enduring wisdom as a foundation for a fulfilling life.

Teaching Ikigai Principles to Children and Adolescents

Raising children in today's fast-paced world comes with its own set of challenges. As guardians of the next generation, it's our responsibility to equip young minds with the tools they need to not just survive, but thrive. One such powerful tool is the concept of *Ikigai*. Instilling the principles of Ikigai in children and adolescents can pave the way for a life filled with purpose and joy. But how do we go about this mission?

It starts with understanding the unique elements of Ikigai and presenting them in ways that resonate with young hearts and minds.

Firstly, it's crucial to simplify the core tenets of Ikigai. While adults might grasp the intersection of passion, profession, vocation, and mission, kids need something more tangible. Start by encouraging them to explore and identify what they love. Whether it's painting, coding, dancing, or simply playing outside, nurture that passion. Remember, passions can ignite into the flames of dreams, and dreams shape futures. Show them that what they love can have a concrete place in their everyday lives and potentially, their future careers.

As children grow, they naturally begin to comprehend that their actions affect the world around them. This is the perfect time to introduce them to the idea that what they love can meet the needs of others. Encourage them to think about how their hobbies or skills might be used to help people, their friends, or even their community. Whether it's writing stories that inspire others, or inventing gadgets that make life easier, kids can start linking their passions to purpose at a tender age.

We live in a society that often equates financial success with self-worth, but Ikigai offers a broader perspective. It's important to guide young minds to understand that while income is essential, it's not the only measure of success. Show them that when you merge what you love with what the world needs, it can also lead to financial stability. Encourage fields and activities that hold economic potential, but always frame it within the context of joy and fulfillment, not just a paycheck.

Children grow from opportunities to showcase what they're good at. Recognize and celebrate their strengths, whether it's a knack for numbers, an ear for music, or an eye for art. The joy of mastering a skill is a key component of Ikigai. This isn't just about boosting their confidence; it's about reinforcing the belief that everyone has something special to offer. Empower them with the mindset that their unique talents can make a mark in the world.

Furthermore, the Ikigai mindset thrives in an atmosphere of continual learning and curiosity. Encourage children to ask questions, pursue knowledge beyond the classroom, and see every difficulty as a learning opportunity. This curiosity will serve them well, enriching their understanding and appreciation for diverse paths and experiences. Instilling a love for learning early on will help them remain adaptable adults, well-equipped for the rapid pace of change the future holds.

Teaching children to live intentionally with Ikigai involves creating habits that reflect their values and interests. Show them how to set small, achievable goals based on their passions and interests. It might be completing a simple project, learning a new skill, or contributing to a group task. Celebrate each milestone, no matter how small. Over time, these "wins" build a narrative of accomplishment and purpose.

Let us not overlook the importance of community and relationships in the journey of Ikigai. Children should be encouraged to build supportive networks among their peers and foster meaningful relationships. Participation in group activities or clubs can teach them valuable skills in teamwork and empathy, showing them how their Ikigai can be experienced and shared, not just pursued in isolation.

Finally, young people should be reminded that life's journey is filled with challenges and changes. Resilience and adaptability are key. They must know that setbacks are not failures but stepping stones to their true purpose. Through stories, discussions, and examples from your own life, help them understand that growth often comes from facing challenges head-on.

Teaching Ikigai to children and adolescents is not about imposing a rigid framework on them; it's about opening up possibilities. It's an invitation to explore life's richness and find the spark that lights their way. By weaving the principles of Ikigai into their fabric of understanding, we're not just preparing them for the future; we're equipping them to shape it with joy and purpose.

Shaping a Future with Purpose and Joy

In a world that's constantly evolving, shaping a future brimming with purpose and joy isn't just a desire—it's a necessity. We live in a time where young souls face unprecedented pressures, from social expectations to academic hurdles, and the digital noise that bombards them daily. It's crucial, now more than ever, to empower them with tools that help them navigate these challenges with confidence and optimism.

Ikigai, the Japanese concept of finding one's reason for being, offers a profound framework for the next generation. It's not just a notion steeped in cultural tradition but a transformative lens through which young people can view their potential. By embracing ikigai, we gift them a compass that doesn't point due north but to their true north—the unique intersection of what they love, what they're good at, what the world needs, and what they can be compensated for.

Nurturing young minds to discover their ikigai starts with curiosity. We must encourage a culture of questioning, where the quest for knowledge and understanding isn't confined to textbooks but born from a genuine love of learning. Imagine a classroom where each question posed is a stepping stone to self-discovery, leading students to uncover passions they never knew existed. That's the kind of environment that fosters true joy and a sense of purpose.

But how do we foster this environment? It begins with reimagining education. Formal education often emphasizes grading and results, but what if it also focused on nurturing individual values and strengths? Schools could incorporate mentorship programs where students learn directly from those already treading their path of purpose. Such interactions can be enlightening, offering a glimpse into the myriad ways one can contribute meaningfully to the world.

Equally important is the role of the community. Communities that foster strong, intergenerational bonds offer youth a well-rounded support system. When young individuals see purpose reflected in the diverse lives of those around them, it shapes their understanding of the many ways they can lead purposeful lives. Grandparents sharing stories of their own ikigai can impart wisdom that textbooks simply can't provide, while parents modeling work-life harmony can illustrate balance in a tangible way.

Incorporating rituals into daily life can also play a pivotal role in shaping a future filled with purpose and joy. Rituals provide a sense of structure and predictability, grounding young people amidst the chaos of everyday life. These rituals needn't be grand; they can be as simple as a morning gratitude practice or a nightly reflection on daily achievements and lessons learned. Over time, such routines can strengthen the intention to live with purpose, making the pursuit of ikigai a natural part of life.

It's not enough, however, to merely talk about these concepts—action is paramount. Encouraging participation in community service can be a doorway for young people to understand their impact on the world around them. Through service, they learn empathy, compassion, and the direct results of their contributions, understanding firsthand how purposeful work brings joy not only to others but to themselves.

We also need to address the digital landscapes where young people spend much of their time. While digital platforms can be overwhelming, they also offer unparalleled opportunities to create and share one's purpose on a global scale. Guiding them to use these tools mindfully can empower young minds to broadcast their passions, connect with like-minded individuals, and even create movements that propel societal change. Teaching digital literacy is as vital as fostering emotional intelligence, ensuring their engagement online is healthy and purposeful.

In conclusion, the journey to shaping a future infused with purpose and joy hinges on making the principles of ikigai accessible and relatable. It involves teaching our youth not only to find joy in their successes but to see setbacks as opportunities for growth. It invites them to continually ask themselves profound questions, to adapt as they evolve, and to embrace the fulfillment that arises from a life well-lived. By instilling these values, we lay the foundation for a generation that doesn't just dream of a better world but actively shapes it.

The key lies not in dictating a singular path but in opening a multitude of possibilities, steering youths toward their inherent potentials. In this way, they grow into individuals who define success not by external accolades but by internal satisfaction—by joy, passion, and the enduring legacy of purpose.

CHAPTER 12:
EVOLVING YOUR IKIGAI

As you reach this pivotal stage in your journey, it's essential to recognize that your ikigai isn't a static destination but a dynamic path that shifts as you grow. Embracing the ever-changing nature of your personal purpose involves flexibility and openness to new experiences and passions. Perhaps you've noticed subtle shifts in your interests or external circumstances pushing you towards new opportunities. These transitions aren't just inevitable—they're vital for fostering resilience and continuous renewal. By preparing for these changes, you align more closely with your evolving sense of self, allowing greater fulfillment and joy in each phase of life. Remember, the art of recalibrating your ikigai is about courageously stepping forward, guided by the wisdom gained through experience and the promise of what lies ahead.

The Ever-Changing Nature of Personal Purpose

Life is a dynamic tapestry of experiences, constantly woven by the choices we make, the lessons we learn, and the dreams we dare to chase. Within this ever-flowing stream, the notion of personal purpose—our ikigai—takes on a similarly fluid nature. It is not fixed; rather, it bends and sways like a reed in the wind, responding to the currents of our existence. To embrace this idea is to embrace life itself, in all its unpredictable beauty.

Understanding that personal purpose can change is liberating. It frees us from the confines of a predetermined path and invites us to explore our lives with curiosity and openness. As human beings, we grow with every experience, and our views, desires, and capabilities shift over time. Holding onto a rigid sense of purpose would be like trying to hold on to sand; the more tightly we grip, the more it slips through our fingers.

The first seeds of personal purpose might be sown in our early years, sparked by childhood dreams or familial inspirations, but these seeds require nurturing. Through adolescence, as we learn more about ourselves and the world, our understanding of what truly matters evolves. The purpose we find in our twenties may not necessarily serve us in our thirties or forties, and that's okay. Our journey is uniquely our own, enriched by change rather than hindered by it.

Consider the artist who starts their career with a passion for capturing landscapes on canvas. As years pass, they might discover a new calling in teaching art to children, finding deeper fulfillment in inspiring others rather than solely creating. The central theme here is not abandoning one for another; it's a transition nurtured by life's experiences, transforming the artist's ikigai into something even more profound.

Seasons of life bring different opportunities and challenges. Graduating from school, starting a family, changing careers, or experiencing loss—each phase reshapes who we are and, correspondingly, what gives our lives meaning. This isn't about inconsistency; it's about alignment. Each new version of ourselves requires a recalibration of what makes us feel alive and purposeful.

At times, external influences can prompt a reevaluation of our purpose. A global crisis, for example, might shift our focus from professional achievements to communal contributions. In the wake of significant natural or personal events, we often find ourselves revisiting old ideologies, questioning past ambitions, and crafting fresh objectives with renewed vigor.

The drive to explore and understand different aspects of one's ikigai doesn't merely arise from necessity; it emerges from an inherent desire to stay engaged with life's offerings. This exploration is akin to tending a garden—constant care and attention allow for flourishing growth.

For some, personal purpose may involve repeated cycles of reinvention. Think of those who thrive on change, the entrepreneurs who shift industries, or the professionals who pivot careers multiple times. Their ikigai thrives precisely because it embraces novelty and transformation, seeing endless opportunities rather than insurmountable obstacles.

Yet, the ever-evolving nature of personal purpose does not mean abandoning what grounds us. Our core values act like a compass, providing direction even as we navigate new terrains. As purpose shifts, these values ensure that our journey stays true to what fundamentally matters to us, offering a sense of continuity amid change.

It's important to recognize that evolution of purpose doesn't always mean moving forward or upwards in a conventional sense. Sometimes, it involves stepping back, reassessing, or even simplifying life. There's profound growth in learning to find fulfillment in the everyday and appreciating the small, seemingly mundane aspects of life that we often overlook.

Accepting the changing nature of personal purpose invites a deeper connection with ourselves and our environment. It calls us to be present, to listen to our inner voice, and to trust it to guide us through life's labyrinthine paths. In doing so, we honor both who we were and who we are becoming.

This fluidity is not a loss, but a gain. Each iteration of our purpose builds upon the last, creating a rich tapestry of experiences and insights unique to our own life story. It teaches resilience, adaptability, and, more importantly, the courage to face the unknown with grace and eagerness.

As you navigate your own journey of ikigai, remember that the key is not to find a static answer, but to engage with an ongoing inquiry. Explore, experiment, and reflect across the different chapters of your life, recognizing that your personal purpose is a living entity—ever changing, and ever yours.

Preparing for Transitions and New Passions

Life is a series of transitions, each bringing new opportunities to rediscover and rekindle your ikigai. Embracing change isn't just about finding new passions; it's also about the courage to let go of what no longer serves you. As you stand at these crossroads, listen to the quiet whisper of curiosity that urges you forward. Ask yourself, "What ignites my spirit at this moment in time?" This isn't a question with a single answer, but rather an invitation to evolve. By welcoming change with open arms, we allow ourselves to grow beyond our self-imposed limitations, propelling us toward new adventures and unexplored passions. Remember, the essence of ikigai is fluid; what serves as your guiding star today may evolve as you gain new experiences and insights. Approach these transitions with an open heart and the understanding that each step, no matter how uncertain, is a testament to your resilience and ever-expanding capacity for joy and fulfillment.

Online Review Request for This Book As you embark on the journey of preparing for transitions and new passions, your feedback on the insights and guidance provided in this book will help others discover the vitality of evolving their own ikigai, so please share your thoughts in an online review to inspire fellow seekers.

THE IKIGAI LEGACY

As we conclude our exploration of ikigai, it's clear that this concept is more than just an intersection of four areas—it's a compass guiding us toward a life rich in purpose and fulfillment. The ancient wisdom encapsulated in ikigai isn't merely theoretical; it is a lived experience, a palpable energy that drives individuals to wake up each morning with joy and determination.

The legacy of ikigai is a call to action. It's about taking the principles we've explored and integrating them into our daily lives. When you embrace your ikigai, you're not just pursuing personal happiness; you're contributing to a ripple effect that extends to your family, your community, and the world at large. Imagine a world where each person acts from a place of passion, aligned with their true purpose—such a world would indeed be transformative.

One of the key takeaways from our journey through ikigai is the importance of intentionality. Living with intention doesn't mean having every moment of your day meticulously planned. Rather, it suggests a consistent commitment to aligning your actions with your deepest values. This approach enables you to weather life's storms with resilience and to celebrate its joys with a heart full of gratitude.

In today's fast-paced world, it's easy to lose sight of what truly matters. Work demands, social commitments, and the ceaseless bombardment of information can obscure our path. Yet, ikigai encourages us to pause, reflect, and reorient ourselves toward being present. By doing so, we forge a legacy that's not just about what we do, but about how we make others feel and the lives we touch along the way.

Community and connection play a quintessential role in the ikigai legacy. As we've discussed, surrounding yourself with a supportive network can enhance your journey toward discovering and living your purpose. Whether through collaborations, friendships, or familial bonds, the strength of community sustains us. It reminds us that we are not alone in our quest for meaning, and that our contributions to the world benefit greatly from collective wisdom.

Furthermore, many of us will find that our ikigai evolves over time. Life is not static—our passions shift, our skills expand, and our needs change. Embracing this evolution is crucial. Instead of clinging to a fixed idea of purpose, understanding that adaptability is a strength can lead to new and exciting pathways. The willingness to adapt keeps our minds sharp, our spirits resilient, and our hearts open to novel possibilities.

In the legacy of ikigai, there is a profound respect for the individual's journey. We each have a unique path, shaped by our experiences, dreams, and choices. However, the essence of ikigai transcends individual pursuits, encouraging us to act as stewards of a larger, more connected world. Let this legacy inspire you to leave not just footprints, but a trail of hope and positivity for future generations.

As we part ways here, remember that the journey of ikigai is ongoing. It invites you to be curious, to question, and to continually seek the intersections of passion, mission, vocation, and profession that create your distinct ikigai. These intersections are dynamic, sometimes requiring recalibration, but always leading you toward a deeper understanding of your life's purpose.

The true beauty of the ikigai legacy lies in its simplicity and depth. In a world that often seeks complexity, ikigai reminds us that the core of a meaningful life is rooted in simple truths: engage with what you love, contribute to what the world needs, be open to change, and cherish the connections with those around you. By following these tenets, we can cultivate a life of substantive fulfillment.

May the lessons of ikigai empower you to live a life with clarity and purpose. As you continue your personal journey, let the legacy of ikigai be your guide, reminding you of the potential each day holds when it begins with intention and ends with reflection. Embrace the journey with an open heart, and may your ikigai light the path forward.

APPENDIX A:
EXERCISES TO DISCOVER YOUR
IKIGAI

Your journey towards finding your ikigai is a deeply personal one. It's about peeling back the layers of your daily existence to uncover the core driving force that gives your life meaning. Here are some exercises designed to guide you as you embark on this transformative quest. These exercises can help you explore different facets of your life and encourage deep reflection on your passions, strengths, and contributions.

1. Reflect on Joyful Moments

Think of times when you've felt truly alive. When were you most enthusiastic, engaged, and satisfied? Make a list of these moments, and identify common themes or activities. These often point towards what you love and are passionate about. Spend some time writing about these experiences, focusing on the feelings they evoked and the aspects that sparked joy.

2. Identify Your Strengths

We all have unique talents and skills. To discover yours, try listing what you're naturally good at. If you're unsure, consider asking friends, family, or colleagues for feedback. Reflect on what tasks or challenges you excel at and consider how these strengths can be further developed and applied in meaningful ways.

3. Clarify Your Values

Your values are the guiding principles that shape your decisions and actions. Write down a list of values that resonate with you, such as honesty, creativity, or compassion. Consider how these values align with your daily life and whether there's a gap between your current situation and what you value most. This awareness can help direct you toward a more aligned and purposeful existence.

4. Explore Your Contributions

One's sense of purpose often emerges from the impact they can have on the world. Think about what contributions you can make to your community or society. This doesn't need to be grand or world-changing; even small acts of kindness and service can reflect your ikigai. Consider volunteer opportunities or projects that align with causes you're passionate about.

5. Envision Your Perfect Day

Take a moment to imagine what a perfect day in your life would look like, from morning till night. What activities fill your time? Who are you with? What routines and rituals give you peace and joy? This exercise not only reveals your passions and interests but also provides insight into the lifestyle that best supports your ikigai.

6. Set Small, Intentional Goals

Break down the large concept of ikigai into smaller, manageable goals that you can integrate into your daily life. Whether it's dedicating more time to hobbies, improving a skill, or fostering relationships, these goals should reflect aspects of your ikigai and help bring you closer to living a balanced, fulfilled life.

7. Engage in Mindful Reflection

Regularly take time to reflect on your progress and adjustments needed on your ikigai journey. This practice should be introspective and free of judgment. Use journaling, meditation, or quiet contemplation as tools to connect with your inner self and ensure you are moving in the direction of purpose and happiness.

Discovering your ikigai isn't a finite task but an ongoing journey of exploration and growth. By consciously engaging with these exercises and embracing the process, you'll uncover the delicate balance between what you love, what you're good at, what the world needs, and what you can be compensated for. This understanding will act as your compass toward a life brimming with purpose and fulfillment.

APPENDIX B:
RESOURCES FOR FURTHER
EXPLORATION

Embarking on the journey to discover your personal ikigai is profoundly transformative. It's a path enriched by the wisdom of those who have explored it before you. Here, I've gathered a selection of resources that can illuminate your path and deepen your understanding. Whether you're seeking books, online communities, or educational courses, these recommendations aim to inspire and support your quest for a purposeful life.

1. Books and Literature

- **"Ikigai: The Japanese Secret to a Long and Happy Life" by Héctor García and Francesc Miralles** - A comprehensive exploration of ikigai, blending philosophical insights with practical advice.

- **"The Blue Zones: 9 Lessons for Living Longer From the People Who've Lived the Longest" by Dan Buettner** - While not solely about ikigai, it delves into the lifestyles that contribute to longevity, often overlapping with ikigai principles.

- **"Drive: The Surprising Truth About What Motivates Us" by Daniel H. Pink** - Offers insights into human motivation that align with finding what drives your ikigai.

2. Online Courses and Lectures

- **Coursera and edX** - These platforms offer numerous courses related to personal development, psychology, and fulfillment that can aid in understanding your ikigai.

- **TED Talks** - Engaging lectures by thought leaders that cover a variety of topics related to passion, purpose, and well-being.

3. Workshops and Retreats

- **Mindfulness Retreats** - Consider attending a retreat that focuses on mindfulness and self-discovery, which often integrate exercises to explore personal purpose.

- **Local Ikigai Workshops** - Look for community events or workshops that focus on ikigai and personal development. These gatherings can provide both knowledge and community support.

4. Online Communities and Forums

- **Reddit: r/ikigai** - Join discussions with a community that shares insights and experiences related to finding one's ikigai.

- **Quora** - Engage with thought-provoking questions and answers about living a life filled with purpose.

5. Podcasts and Audio Resources

- **"The Tim Ferriss Show"** - Known for its diverse guests and topics, including discussions on finding fulfillment and motivation.

- **"The Tony Robbins Podcast"** - Offers motivational insights that align with personal growth and discovering purpose.

Your exploration doesn't end here. Each resource can lead to new discoveries and personal revelations. Remember, the journey to a more fulfilling life is lifelong, marked by continuous learning and adaptation. Embrace these resources as companions on your path to living with purpose, joy, and a deeper sense of meaning.